So you want to be a medical mum?

So you want to be a medical mum?

A guide for female medics who have ever thought that maybe, somehow, one day, they might want to have a baby

Dr Emma Hill

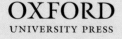
OXFORD
UNIVERSITY PRESS

OXFORD
UNIVERSITY PRESS

Great Clarendon Street, Oxford OX2 6DP

Oxford University Press is a department of the University of Oxford.
It furthers the University's objective of excellence in research, scholarship,
and education by publishing worldwide in

Oxford New York

Auckland Cape Town Dar es Salaam Hong Kong Karachi
Kuala Lumpur Madrid Melbourne Mexico City Nairobi
New Delhi Shanghai Taipei Toronto

With offices in

Argentina Austria Brazil Chile Czech Republic France Greece
Guatemala Hungary Italy Japan Poland Portugal Singapore
South Korea Switzerland Thailand Turkey Ukraine Vietnam

Oxford is a registered trade mark of Oxford University Press
in the UK and in certain other countries

Published in the United States
by Oxford University Press Inc., New York

A catalogue record for this title is available from the British Library
Data available

Library of Congress Cataloging in Publication Data
Data available

Typeset by Cepha Imaging Private Ltd., Bangalore, India
Printed in Great Britain
on acid-free paper by
Ashford Colour Press Ltd., Gosport, Hampshire, UK

ISBN 978-0-19-923758-6

10 9 8 7 6 5 4 3 2 1

Whilst every effort has been made to ensure that the contents of this book
are as complete, accurate and-up-to-date as possible at the date of writing.
Oxford University Press is not able to give any guarantee or assurance that
such is the case. Readers are urged to take appropriately qualified medical
advice in all cases. The information in this book is intended to be useful to
the general reader, but should not be used as a means of self-diagnosis or
for the prescription of medication.

Thanks

I am eternally grateful to the wonderful medical mums (and dads) who gave their time to contribute to this book. Over 60 doctors and medical students were involved, and many gave their spare time in the evenings or at weekends, in order to talk to me. About three-quarters of those doctors have small children under the age of 5, and they were invaluable in giving an insight into what it is like being a medic and a parent. Many opened their hearts and talked at length about their experiences, both good and bad, allowing their innermost secrets to be shared with the readers of this book. I thank you, on behalf of myself, and on behalf of those who will hopefully turn to this book for advice and guidance. Thank you to the medical mums who supplied photos, and thanks also to the non-medics who contributed with their opinions.

My thanks must also go to Fiona and Chris, at Oxford University Press, for giving me the opportunity to write this book; thanks for taking me seriously when you first read my proposal, and for your help along the way.

I wouldn't be sitting here writing this book if it wasn't for my wonderful girlfriends. Iris is so lucky to have her fabulous aunties, and if she grows up like any of you I'll be so proud. For the visits and phone calls in the early days, when the going was a bit tough, you were amazing; especially Lis, Charlotte, Jane, Harriet, and Carole. Hannah, Natasa, and Dee, her lovely aunties too. Lou, you rock. Sophie, I've said it before and I'll say it again, how can I say thank you enough; you saved my life. And Abi, the most wonderful friend that anyone could wish for, you're simply the best.

To the NCT girls; Nicole, Ali, Lorna, Sheetal, Clarissa, and Helen. How amazing that I could have found such special friendships at this time in my life. Your kindness when Iris was born, and to this day, will always be appreciated. Thanks must also go to my newfound friends in Hackney, especially Jude and Vicky, who have been fabulously supportive.

Without the help of last minute babysitters, this book couldn't have existed; Bias, our favourite Wicked Uncle, and Joyce, from next door. Maria Deering, our fantastic childminder, has enabled me to return to work with confidence; you're priceless, and we're very lucky to have found you.

I'd like to thank my programme directors, Phil and Sarah; Sarah, for your help with the book, and your encouragement, and Phil, for not killing me whenever I announced I was pregnant/going part time/about to be unemployed/going full time, and generally messing up your rotas. Thank you.

Jack, who encouraged me from embryonic medical student to fully fledged doctor; I can never thank you enough. To Helen Stoney, another great friend, who also encouraged me to work hard and aim for the stars.

Thanks to my mum and dad, for accepting that I would never do anything in life in the proper, conventional, manner. Thank you for supporting me, in more ways than one, through medical school and beyond, and for helping out with childcare. Thanks to GG, the best great grandma in the world, and to my in-laws, for giving me a husband that doesn't need waiting on hand and foot.

Finally, thanks to Euan, for being my hero, my lover and my best friend. For being there for better and for worse, in sickness and in health, and all the amazing times we've had with our beautiful girl. I love you.

All the photos in the book are of children who have medical mums—thanks to all those who supplied pictures.

This book is for Euan and Iris.

Preface

I spent years wondering when and how to have children; it seemed an impossible task as a doctor. When I found out that I was pregnant, only 6 months into my career, I was delighted. But I had no one to turn to for advice, and could find no written sources of support. How would I manage my shifts later on in the pregnancy? How much time should I take off? What would it be like, coming back to work with a baby to care for? My colleagues and friends were only too happy to talk about it though, and I soon discovered that there were endless unanswered questions for medical women.

I was pregnant as a junior house officer (FY1) in surgery, and then as a senior house officer (FY2) in health care of the elderly. I took some time off after I'd had my baby, and came back part time for a year; then I returned full time. In every job, I've been bombarded by questions; people wondering how and when to have their families, and how to continue working once there's a child or two at home.

With this in mind, I set out to pool the untapped resources of the real experts; the medical mums. Going through pregnancy, and being a new mum, had taught me so much, and I knew that others would feel the same. By talking to doctors and medical students who had also had children, for their advice and experiences, I was able to start writing this book. Along with supplying factual information that was hard to find, (such as on maternity leave,) I have hopefully created a very rough guide to having it all; wonderful children, and a fabulous career. Good luck!

Glossary and abbreviations

AML	Additional Maternity Leave
Banding	Pay structure according to anti-social hours
Bleep	Device designed to drive you mad; a pager
BMA	British Medical Association
CCST	Certificate of Completion of Specialist Training
CIS	Children's Information Service
Consultant	The boss, in terms of hospital medicine
CT	Computed tomography scan
CTC	Child Tax Credit
CTG	Cardiotocograph; a record of fetal heart rate and rhythm
DTI	Department of Trade and Industry
EDD	Estimated Delivery Date
EOC	Equal Opportunities Commission
EPAU	Early pregnancy assessment unit
FHSA	Family Health Service Authority
GMC	General Medical Council
GP	General Practitioner
GP Registrar	GP in training (now ST3 general practice)
Grand Round	Presentation or teaching session for medical staff
HMRC	Her Majesties Revenue and Customs
HR	Human Resources
HSE	Health and Safety Executive
HV	Health Visitor
ITU	Intensive care unit
IVF	In Vitro Fertilization
Locum	Temporary appointment
MA	Maternity Allowance
MAU	Medical Admission Unit
MD	Doctor of Medicine
MDU	Medical Defence Union
MMC	Modernizing Medical Careers
MRC ...	Member of the Royal College of ... e.g. physicians/surgeons

NCT	National Childbirth Trust
NICE	National Institute for Clinical Excellence
Number	Training number; meant you could train to consultant level
OOH	Out of Hours
OML	Ordinary Maternity Leave
PCT	Primary Care Trust
PhD	Doctor of philosophy
Physician	Medical doctor
PR	via the rectum
PRHO	Pre-Registration House Officer (now foundation year 1)
QOF	Quality and Outcomes Framework
RCGP	Royal College of General Practitioners
Registrar	Reg/Specialist registrar ... One below a consultant
SCBU	Special care baby unit
SHO	Senior House Officer (junior hospital doctor)
SMP	Statutory Maternity Pay
SPP	Statutory Paternity Pay
TENS	Transcutaneous electrical nerve stimulation
UCAS	Universities and Colleges Admissions Service
WTC	Working Tax Credit
VTS	Vocational Training Scheme for general practice

Medical specialities: a quick guide for the non-medic

A&E	Accident and Emergency
Anaesthetics	Inducing sleep or sedation for surgery, monitoring recovery; also involves protecting the breathing apparatus in trauma and other seriously ill patients
Dermatology	Skin diseases
Diabetology	Diabetes (high blood sugar)
Endocrinology	Hormones, such as sex hormones, thyroid, growth hormones
ENT	Ear, nose and throat
Gastroenterology	Gastrointestinal disease, including the digestive tract, the liver, and pancreas
Geriatrics	Care of older people (determined by either age or needs)
GP	General practice

Haematology	Disorders of the blood and blood-forming tissues
ICU	Intensive care; for very sick patients
Infectious diseases	Diseases that are infectious, transmitted from one person to another
MaxFax	Maxillofacial; the region of the face, jaws, and related structures
Nephrology	Deals with diseases of the kidneys
Neurology	Nerves, brain, and spinal cord disorders
Obs & Gynae	Childbirth and reproduction
Ophthalmology	Eyes
Orthopaedics	A surgical speciality dealing with disorders of bones and joints
Pathology	The study of disease processes, involving tissue samples from living patients or dead people
Paediatrics	Children
Plastics	Plastic surgery
Psychiatry	The speciality that deals with mental illness
Radiology	X-rays and scans, ultrasounds, other imaging and the interpretation of
Renal	A branch of medicine dealing with kidney disease
Respiratory	Chest medicine (the lungs)
Rheumatology	Joints, tendons, muscles, and ligaments
Surgery	Treatment or management by operation
Urology	Diseases of the urinary tract

Hospital hierarchy

In the old days
- Medical student
- Pre Registration House Officer (PRHO), also called House Officers
- Senior House Officer (SHO)
- Registrar/Specialist Registrar (SpR)
- Consultant

Nowadays
- Medical student
- Foundation Year (FY) 1 and 2
- Specialist Training (ST) 1–X
- Consultant

A note about Modernizing Medical Careers (MMC)

At the time of being interviewed for this book, many of the doctors were Senior House Officers (SHOs) or Registrars. In August 2007, the training grades of doctors (after their Foundation Years) were changed to Specialist Training (ST). It was extremely difficult to convert SHO and Registrar levels to the equivalent ST level, i.e. 1, 2, 3; for the purposes of this book, all quotes from doctors between Foundation Years and Consultant are simply labelled as ST, plus the speciality.

A note about economics

Prices go up, and rates of benefits change. All the payments and prices quoted in the book were correct at the time of writing (July 2007) but undoubtedly things will differ over time.

Contents

Introduction

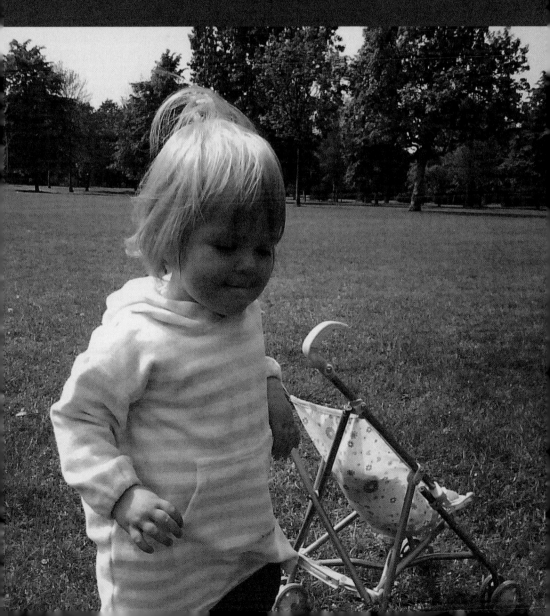

'Oh dear,' said the consultant, 'was it a mistake?' I held my breath and fixed a smile on my face, prepared to repeat the mantra that had now become as familiar as my bleep number. 'No, it wasn't a mistake, not at all. A little earlier than we expected, yes … But a wonderful surprise all the same. Thanks.'

Why was being a pregnant junior doctor such a curiosity? I was a normal, healthy female going through a normal life experience. Over time, I had encountered some doctors from a separate evolutionary pathway, yet no one batted an eyelid at their weirdness. Suddenly I was feeling like a minor celebrity, or at least the baby was, besieged by questions of 'How?' and 'Why now?'

Most people were incredibly supportive. My friends at work were delighted to have 'their own baby,' and decided on a list of names long before my husband and I had even thought of one. Yet there was no denying the fact that pregnant doctors were thin on the ground at my hospital, or were at the very least in hiding. However, over 60% of graduates in medicine in the UK are now female, and most will, at some point in their careers, decide to have a baby or two. So where do they all go? Do they, like migratory animals, disappear to other places to reproduce, or wait until they are GPs or consultants? Certainly, most doctors seem to wait until they have reached a particular point in their career path before they decide to have a family. But the numbers of mature female medical students is increasing year by year, and one can only assume that in the future pregnant doctors will be familiar throughout all grades.

We might think that it's hard work being a medical mum, but women in medicine have never had it so good. I don't want this book to be a rant about female doctors and the presence or absence of the glass ceiling, but doctors whose children are now grown up can tell younger medics a story or two. When they were pregnant, women formed a smaller percentage of doctors, and there was often not the option of working part time. Nowadays, doctors work fewer hours even when full time, and they can work less than full time in most fields of medicine. Professor Yvonne Carter, who is one of only three women ever to be appointed as Dean of a medical school in the UK, was a busy inner city GP when she had her son, in the 1980s. Professor Parveen Kumar, author of one of the most well recognized medical textbooks (and former President of the British Medical Association) had her daughters while she was training in the male dominated world of gastroenterology in the seventies.

I met my husband, Michael Bannon, in 1986, when I was working on the GP Vocational Training Scheme in Liverpool, and was doing a six month rotation at Alder Hey Children's Hospital. I was an SHO, and Mike was a registrar in paediatrics. We started going out when I was doing my GP Registrar year a few months later, and was revising for the Diploma in Child Health … I asked him to give me a tutorial on paediatric murmurs, and I'm still waiting for that tutorial!

We were married in 1988, and lots of my patients came [to the service], because I was a GP principal in Liverpool by then. I discovered I was pregnant a few days before our first wedding anniversary. I worked full time, and it was a very busy urban practice … It was the kind of practice where you might do sixteen visits a day, and we did our own out of hours work at night and weekends. I was the usual 'not a very good doctor as a patient', and went to my antenatal appointments at lunch time and didn't take time off in the daytime to go and attend antenatal classes, but I went to NCT classes with Mike at night.

Because I was a GP Principal, it was the 'good old days', when you were responsible for finding your own maternity locum … Also the money that you received then from the FHSA didn't cover the actual locum costs, and in my practice agreement it said that I had to meet that difference myself. I took 13 weeks maternity leave, which was the standard in general practice at the time, but I'd saved up two weeks holiday, so technically I was going to have 15 weeks off.

I worked until 36 weeks and Christopher was born two weeks later just after Christmas … It was a difficult delivery, which wasn't easy with my husband being a paediatrician, thinking he was going to have to resuscitate his own baby. I then had 13 weeks off with him, and went back to work on the 1st April 1990 … I remember it because it was the day that the new GP contract was implemented!

I went back to the practice full time, and had a full time nanny during the week who didn't 'live in', who I'd actually heard about on the grapevine through a patient at the practice … When I came back to work, my husband was starting to think about looking for a consultant post, and within a few months, he was appointed to a post in North Staffordshire. It meant I had to stop and take stock of what I wanted to do next, and it gave me a chance to reflect on whether I wanted to continue as a full time GP … Also to think about whether we wanted to continue the arrangement with our nanny. I joined another practice that was still technically full time as a '26 hour' principal, but it was about a third of the work I was doing in Liverpool.

We'd had a long debate [about childcare] and my sister, Alma, came to live with us. She gave up her job, and sold her house, and we put all the money in together and bought a bigger house. She moved in, and was there as a family member and replaced our nanny. So really, since

Christopher was a few months old, she's been doing a lot of the day to day stuff, school runs … And she's the main reason why I've had the opportunity to do a really full on academic role.

When I joined the practice in Newcastle-under-Lyme, [when Christopher was about 10 months old], I also applied for an RCGP research training fellowship, which gave me two sessions of protected research time … I basically did my MD while Christopher was a baby/toddler, and was a research fellow at the University of Keele whilst I was doing that.

Christopher is seventeen now and is considering his own UCAS application and the attraction of a degree in Natural Sciences, and he doesn't want to apply for medicine at the moment. It is a bit sad, because I suppose I was hoping that he'd do it. He grew up as a baby with both of us doing our own on call; we went through a number of years where both of us were doing one in three … So one parent was nearly always on call. Mike and I are both the type of parents who leave at seven in the morning and come back at dinner time, and we often miss sports days and things. So I suppose he's grown up thinking, is that the kind of life he really wants to have? He has said he might apply for graduate entry medicine … But I think we've probably put him off. Maybe we've not been the kind of examples we think we've been. But he's very bright and works hard, he wants to go down an academic route … I'm sure he'll be a professor of something one day!'

Professor Yvonne Carter OBE (Academic General Practitioner and Honorary Consultant in Primary Care, Coventry Teaching PCT; Dean, Warwick Medical School)

When I had my first baby, I had two weeks off … I went off on the Monday, and when I came back two weeks later everyone was asking if I'd had a nice holiday! I was a registrar [in gastroenterology], and I came back full time to a job in the liver unit, which was very busy … When I'd been pregnant, I was lucky enough to have very kind male colleagues, who would offer to do all the radiation work, as a swap for me doing other work for them.

The lady who had looked after me when I was small ended up living near us, and she became our childminder. Before I left for work at 6.45am, I'd put the baby in the carry cot with her nappies and things, drive to the childminder's house and drop the baby off. Then I'd have to drop my husband off at the station, as he was commuting from

London to Brighton to work as a registrar, then I'd go to work. The whole thing had to be repeated in reverse at about 6 or 7pm, and in the end, she decided we all looked so tired; she started to make our evening meal for us too!

When I had my second baby, I took sixteen weeks off, because we were also moving house; my husband [David Leaver] had just secured a consultant post in Epsom. That time off was great, I did things I'd never done before, like sitting around having coffee, and going to the swings.

For the first year or so after going back to work, my mother came over sometimes to help, and my husband and I boxed it and coxed it with our takes ... Then we had nannies. In the end, my daughters decided that they didn't like nannies (the one we had was rather strict), so they wrote an advert for an au pair and put it in the Lady magazine! They were only five and seven at the time ... But we ended up getting an au pair, who stayed with us for five years ... I remember coming home and seeing them sitting having tea with her, and laughing and joking, and realising how happy the girls were.

We decided not to send them away [to Boarding School], as firstly we wanted them to have a decent education, and secondly we wanted to have some sort of impression on them, seeing them at weekends and such. Rachel is 34 now, and Susannah is 32. Susannah is a doctor, and is about to go back to work full time [as a registrar in respiratory medicine] after having six months off to have a baby ... My grandson is gorgeous, and I have to say, it's just fantastic being a grandma! You have no idea how great it is until it happens to you, and I'm probably going to take half-time retirement at the end of August so I can spend more time with him.

In terms of advice to female doctors, I would say that having children and working is always a compromise. But you won't regret any of it. As a girl, you do have to work harder. Of course, it's all different now, but in my day it would be fine for the boys to go off and play golf, but if I announced I was going to go to my daughter's nativity play, it was all 'Oh Parveen, come on ...!' Remember that I was the only woman in the gastro unit for twenty years.

Professor Parveen Kumar CBE (Hon. Consultant Physician and Gastroenterologist; Professor of Clinical Medical Education, Reader in Gastroenterology at St Bartholomew's and the Royal London School of Medicine and Dentistry; President of the British Medical Association, 2007)

Ever since thinking about medicine as a career, I had also wanted to have a family. Despite scouring the bookshops and internet, I could find nothing to encourage me that it was possible. Being a doctor is a demanding job with long hours and a long career path. There are books available for other working mothers; mothers who work in the city, in banking. But I feel that being a doctor is unique, and that pregnancy as a doctor comes with its own challenges. In which other job can you expect to be on your feet for hours on end one day, then sitting in a 6-hour clinic the next? To operate on a patient with hepatitis C while holding on to your bladder for an entire morning? And to be expected to know everything about what's happening to your body, and to know everything about the baby when it's born, even though you've been studying ophthalmology for the last 10 years? And in which other profession do most women seem to have no idea of their rights to leave, pay, and working conditions?

We have fantastic jobs. The system we work in would collapse if we all left once we had children to look after. The challenge is to combine family and work, if that is what we choose to do. For some women that will mean giving up medicine for several years before deciding to return; for others, it will mean going back to work full-time after only a short maternity leave. Each woman has her own unique decision to make, which is right for her and her family at that time.

Whether you choose to have children before medical school, or as a GP or consultant, you will go through an extraordinary life experience. That experience will be shaped by your chosen field, your level of training, your partner and their work, and your family and friends. Your expectations of motherhood, your ambitions at work, and your support at home will all play a part. We will all have moments of doubt, of making difficult decisions between career and family. We will all feel guilty, at one time or another, for putting family or work first. We will share moments of complete exhaustion, while dealing with sick patients at work and sick children at home. But we will have years of indescribable joy with our families. We are all women, in a medical world, trying to be a mother and a doctor. We are striving for a combination of the most challenging, yet rewarding, jobs on offer.

Chapter 1

Before you take the plunge

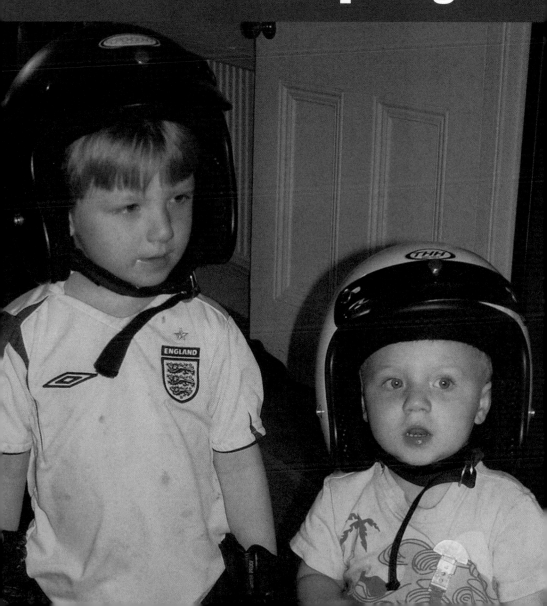

> Don't leave it too late … You might regret that you were never a consultant, but you'll never regret the fact that you've had kids.
>
> *Consultant surgeon*

How do you know when it's the right time to have children? Maybe you'll never know. My mum, who is not a doctor, told me that there would never be a right time in my life. She insisted that women can find a reason not to have children at almost any stage in their career, and that if you try too hard to plan things you could end up close to retirement, still wondering when the right time might be.

> Before I got pregnant, I talked to quite a few doctors, women and men, and they all said don't wait for the right time in your career, or your academic studies or anything, because … It won't come … Just do it if it feels right. Else you'll regret waiting.
>
> *FY1 doctor*

I started medical school when I was 24, having previously done a degree and worked in another profession. Maybe if I had started as a spring chicken, I wouldn't have spent so much time wondering how and when … But I couldn't help it. Was it best to have my children while I was still a student? My hours were very flexible, there were long holidays, and if I had to miss the odd day or two nobody would have noticed; students had managed to slip into a drunken coma for several weeks and get away with it before now. I was broke anyway, so there wasn't the issue of money to worry about, and perhaps I could have tried to study part-time once I'd had the baby. But how long would my medical degree take? It already stretched out in front of me like a never-ending sea of exams and lectures. My graduation year was way off in the future, like talking about the millennium when you were twelve and laughing at how old you'd be when you got there. How on earth would I buy things for the baby, when I was earning just forty five pounds a week as a barmaid? Could a toddler survive on a diet of tinned pilchards on toast, like me and my flat mate? Maybe I'd never make it though, I'd drop out of medicine, because life would be too hard and I wouldn't be taken seriously by the consultants teaching me.

Perhaps I'd better wait until I was a Foundation Year doctor, or a house officer as we were known in those days. If I timed it right, I might even get some maternity pay, and at least I'd have a job to come back to. But how would I cope being pregnant in a busy clinical job, being the bottom of the heap, and trying to crawl up such a steep learning curve at the same time? I'd never met a pregnant house officer, so where were they all? Perhaps they all ended up in a cupboard in the basement of the hospital, exhausted by lack of lunch and computers that didn't work.

> I'd always wanted children quite young. I'd never worked out in my head when to have them, but it's nice in lots of ways [having a baby now] … My friends are in doctor's accommodation with mouse traps

all over the place, but I get home from work to see the baby, and [my partner] has cooked dinner for me!

FY1 doctor

I do feel a bit like an alien being a house officer with a baby … But I just look around me, at all the other doctors going through the motions and being unhappy, and I think come on, what's really important in life?!

FY1 doctor

Doctors who waited until the end of their specialist training; now perhaps they had the right idea. They'd finished their Registrar (ST) posts, and were on the brink of becoming GPs or consultants. They earned a decent salary, and got good maternity pay. They'd passed their important exams for the moment, and had small people called house officers to run around doing jobs for them when they were exhausted. But I would be nearly forty, if my training ran like clockwork, and maybe I didn't want to chance it. I couldn't bear the thought of leaving it too late, and missing out on something that was more important to me than anything work could offer.

I think that people are delaying it until they're older. We were always told 'Oh, have your baby when you're a consultant,' but I think that's wrong … When you're in training, there's always the infantry to come and fill in your space … There's always another piece of cannon fodder that can fill your gap … As a consultant, you'll have a list to do; you can't just not turn up. By delaying it [until you're a consultant] you're too old and your fertility drops, and you could spend four years having IVF before you even get pregnant, so I would always encourage my female trainees to have their babies early.

Consultant colo-rectal surgeon

In medicine, we follow such a structured career path that every doctor who wants a family seems to worry about when they can do it. What is right for one woman is a complete nightmare for another, and a lot will depend on how quickly you want to reach a set stage, be it getting through your Foundation years or waiting until you are a consultant or GP. As a female medic, I think the only way of planning your family (and I use planning in the loosest sense, as this implies we have some sort of control over it) is to decide when you definitely don't want to get pregnant, then use reliable contraception. Working lots of nights when your partner works days is a proven method, but even intelligent women can be tricked by the old wives tale of thinking that it takes ages to get pregnant once you've come off the Pill. Alternatively, you may find yourself trying for years in vain. If only we knew which way things would go.

You have all these plans, and I think particularly as medics we do it, Right, I'm going to do this then this, then this, and then I'll get pregnant by this time ... But in actual fact it may take you ten years to have a child.... I just think, well I'm just planning all of this, but is it going to happen?

ST surgery

My ex-wife, she was a doctor... Oh my god, it was just planning one exam after the other, always busy doing something... Then just when I thought she'd finished with exams, she announces she's doing a PhD... It was like she was always finding excuses not to have kids, she didn't have time.

A male non-medic

Modernizing medical careers (MMC)

In the past, doctors started work as pre-registration house officers (PRHOs). After a year, they became senior house officers (SHOs) for anything up to 4 years or more, then got a national training number (NTN) and became a specialist registrar (SpR).

After successfully completing SpR training, hospital doctors were awarded certificates of completion of specialist training (CCST), and GP registrars were awarded a letter of completion of training. The doctor could then apply for a senior post (consultant or GP).

Under MMC, graduates from medical school apply nationally for the Foundation Programme, which consists of 2 years (FY1 and FY2). They then compete for specialist or GP 'run-through' training programmes. These take about 3 years for general practice, and 5–7 years for other specialities. Unless a doctor is going into an academic medical career, a research degree is not required for application to a specialist or GP training programme.

Doctors who have completed the Foundation programme, but don't go into run-through specialist or GP training, can apply for fixed-term specialist training posts. Posts last for a year, and are only available in hospital settings (they only apply for the first 2 years of training—no posts are offered at the third year of specialist training or beyond).

Having completed their run-through specialist training, the doctor is awarded a Certificate of Completion of Training (CCT), and can then apply for a senior post (consultant or GP).

For further information, go to the MMC website at www.mmc.nhs.uk

I was an SHO, and my partner was also an SHO, we were working in the same hospital. We knew we'd have kids one day ... I'd just found out that I'd passed my Part One's ... I'd failed it the first time; I'd sort of been pushed into it by my boss ... So when I suddenly found out I was pregnant I was really shocked, it wasn't on the cards at all, I didn't know what to do. I was so worried, not about telling my family or anything like that, but about telling my boss, the lead guy ... And when I finally did, all tearful and everything, he said 'Well congratulations, that's great, isn't it?' and I thought well yes, wow, I suppose it is, and then it all seemed ok!

Consultant renal physician

As a doctor, the most important thing to bear in mind is probably your chosen speciality. In certain fields, such as general practice, my own experience has taught me that you will be treated as a normal human being who is going through a normal life experience. Of course, if you want to be a neurosurgeon, there is (in theory) no reason why you can't have children early on in your career. But you must be aware that you will be competing for jobs against people who can be at work all hours of the day and night and who have no other commitments apart from a houseplant or two (and those are probably dead). Remember also that unless you work full time, you'll be in a training grade until you're sprouting grey hairs, especially if you did exciting things such as a previous degree or a PhD. But anything is possible if you work hard and are determined. Don't let other people, especially doctors, put you off. If they say you can't do surgery because you're a woman and your life will be miserable, then it probably means that they're miserable in their job. Be realistic, and accept that combining children and medicine is challenging, but always stick to your guns and go for a speciality you enjoy. Never settle for something you feel you 'should' do just because you want to have a family, and never settle for a speciality you don't love just because you think it'll be easier.

Some dermatology departments had all their registrars pregnant at once ... It's a great job to do as a woman, if you want to have a family, people are very understanding.

Consultant dermatologist

A large part of why I did general practice was because I want to have a family ... I wanted to have the chance to stay at home, or work part time, and I knew that would be difficult in a hospital speciality. I wanted my life to be more important than my job.

ST general practice

They hadn't taken on a female [surgical] trainee for ages, and it was a really big deal that I had got the job ... I was so over the moon ... Then about four days into the post, I found out that I was pregnant. It was a complete shock, and I panicked. Actually, in the end, they were great about it.

ST surgery

Table 1 Percentage of female consultants by speciality (Eccles and Sanders, 2008)

Specialty	Percentage of consultants who are female
Accident and emergency medicine	16
Adult psychiatry	23
Anaesthetics	25
Audiological medicine	45
Breast surgery/surgical oncology	10
Cardiology	6
Cardiothoracic surgery	3
Care of the elderly	14
Chemical pathology	10
Child and adolescent psychiatry	43
Clinical genetics	4
Clinical oncology	40
Clinical pharmacology	5
Coloproctology and upper GI surgery	11
Dermatology	30
Endocrine and diabetes	8
ENT surgery	10–15
Family planning and reproductive healthcare	91
Forensic pathology	10
Gastroenterology	10
General practice	30
Genito-Urinary medicine	19
Haematology	28
Histopathology and cytopathology	29
Maxillofacial surgery	0.5
Medical oncology	13
Microbiology	33
Neurology	12
Neurosurgery	5

So you want to be a medical mum?

Table 1   Percentage of female consultants by speciality (Eccles and Sanders, 2008)—cont'd

Specialty	Percentage of consultants who are female
Nuclear medicine	25
Obstetrics and gynaecology	20
Old age psychiatry	27
Ophthalmology	12
Orthopaedic surgery	1
Paediatric surgery	4
Paediatrics	35
Palliative medicine	50
Plastic surgery	5
Psychiatry of learning disability	30
Public health medicine	38
Radiology	24
Respiratory medicine	9
Rheumatology	20
Transfusion medicine	60
Trauma surgery	1
Urology	10
Vascular surgery	1
Virology	44

I was working with a part time diabetologist, who said 'Well you should try something like rheumatology part time, it's all you can expect really, as a working mother.'

Consultant renal physician

Specialities with a relatively high proportion of flexible trainees

- Anaesthesia
- General Practice
- Psychiatry
- Paediatrics
- Pathology
- Medical specialities

(Matheson & Biggs, 1994)

When trying to plan their family, most doctors also have to think about money. Despite your mother's insistence that babies are happiest playing with paper bags and old newspaper, you somehow end up spending a small fortune on them, and the fact that you're not at work adds to the financial hiccup. The problem with waiting until you're earning more is that you can easily spend time putting it off as you gather speed up the career ladder, only to realize that you've got lots of money but can't get pregnant years down the line. Important things to bear in mind are issues around maternity leave and pay (see Chapter 8), as you'll be kicking yourself if you find out that you've missed getting maternity pay by a matter of days. Working part time as a junior doctor, even if you can get some out-of-hours funding, doesn't pay very well. If you're the main bread winner of the family, it can be very stressful trying to work flexibly and pay the mortgage. As a consultant or GP, your basic salary is higher, so cutting your hours will make less of a difference overall.

Only slightly less stressful than trying to plan a pregnancy, or pay the mortgage, is trying to get a job. With the onset of MMC, the stress levels have risen to boiling point, and many female medics feel that until they are on a definite career path they cannot even contemplate getting pregnant. As far as the regulations are concerned, you can apply for a job, and attend the job interview, even if you are 'carrying a water-melon.' You cannot be discriminated against because you are pregnant. In the real world, however, it can be more than a bit unsettling to go through job applications while pregnant.

Applying for jobs and pregnant?

You can apply for a job at any time in your pregnancy, or when you are on maternity leave. You don't necessarily have to disclose that you're pregnant, especially early on, but if you're over about 25 weeks, then your employer needs to know in order for you to get your maternity leave and pay sorted out.

If your consultant is your referee and knows that you are pregnant, they are not allowed to state it without your permission. Some forms may ask whether there are any 'health issues' about which the panel should know. However, as a pregnant woman you are simply undergoing a normal physiological process, not ill health. To make sure no one is treated unfairly, yourself or your potential employer, it makes sense to get some legal advice.

The easiest way to do this is probably to phone Ask BMA if you are a member, with your referee present, and talk to an advisor; you can make sure neither of you is worried about what to say or do.

Once you know you have the job, you need to inform your employer by about 25 weeks gestation, or sooner if you feel uncomfortable waiting that long (or are huge). Bear in mind that your employer will have to sort out rotas and cover, so letting them know sooner rather than later makes sense.

BMA members can phone Ask BMA: phone 0870 60 60 828
Monday–Friday 8.30 a.m. to 6 p.m.

My wife turned up to the first day at her new job [as a medical registrar] absolutely massive … She'd decided not to tell anyone … I think a few eyebrows were raised, but at the end of the day it was how she wanted to go about it.

ST surgery

Doctors in the armed forces

The Medical Cadetship scheme sponsors medical students for 5 years of their medical training, from the beginning of the third year at medical school until the end of Foundation Year 2. In return, you must serve in the army for 5 years after the end of the FY2 year.

All servicewomen are entitled to 18 weeks Ordinary Maternity Leave (OML), whether they leave the service or return to duty after they've had their baby. Servicewomen who return to duty are also entitled to 30 weeks Occupational Maternity Absence, in addition to the 18 weeks OML. You must return to work no later than 37 weeks from the beginning of the week of childbirth.

The army operates a Confidential Support Line (CSL), a free-phone help-line for soldiers and their dependants. It offers help with equal opportunities, harassment and emotional issues. It operates 7 days a week from 10.30 to 22.30 (UK time).

Contact the CSL on:

- 0800 731 4880 (from the UK)
- 0800 1827 395 (from Germany)
- 800 91065 (from Cyprus)
- Rest of the world: phone 00 44 1980 630854
- http://www.army.mod.uk

I loved being involved in the Military, but I joined the [Territorial Army], instead of going for the army, so I could leave when I wanted to have a family ...

ST surgery

The [Territorial] Army decided to send me to Afghanistan ... They hadn't compulsorily mobilized people since the Korean War. It turned out that we didn't go... My daughter was two, and I would have had to go for six months... It was awful, and I had just two weeks notice, and I cried, and cried... In the end, it was fine, and we didn't go, but I was very angry. And I knew that next, they would send us to Iraq ... By the time the second brown envelope dropped through the door [with my call-up papers], I had literally just got the blue stripe on the pregnancy test. I did do a lot of work at that point, I did a lot of trauma training [with the troops], but obviously I couldn't go... There was one girl, at the airport, on the phone to her daughters... She didn't know when she would next be able to speak to them, if she would be allowed to, if she would even be able to get a signal... She just crumpled, and so did I.

Consultant trauma and orthopaedic surgeon

With all this babble about children, spare a thought for the female medics who don't want to have children, or who can't. The subject of family life, when and how to have children, underlies many seemingly benign conversations over lunch or in the mess. Imagine how it must feel to constantly explain to your colleagues that you've either found yourself unable to get pregnant, or that for whatever reason you've decided that having children is not for you; at one end of the spectrum, the pregnant medical student attracts curiosity because they have done it so soon, and at the other is the female consultant, highly successful, batting off questions about why they haven't done it.

I think people make an assumption, because you're a woman. I've been asked about having children... To be honest, I don't feel strongly either way, it would be up to my partner... So I guess that in terms of moving faster up the career ladder, yes, I think I do have a definite advantage [as a gay doctor] because I won't ever be pregnant, so I can advance more quickly in my career than other women.

ST medicine

References

Eccles E, Sanders S (2008) *So You Want to be a Brain Surgeon* (3rd edn). Oxford University Press, Oxford.

Matheson KH, Biggs JSG (1994) Outcome of flexible training in East Anglian region. *BMJ* 1994; **309**(6946) 29.

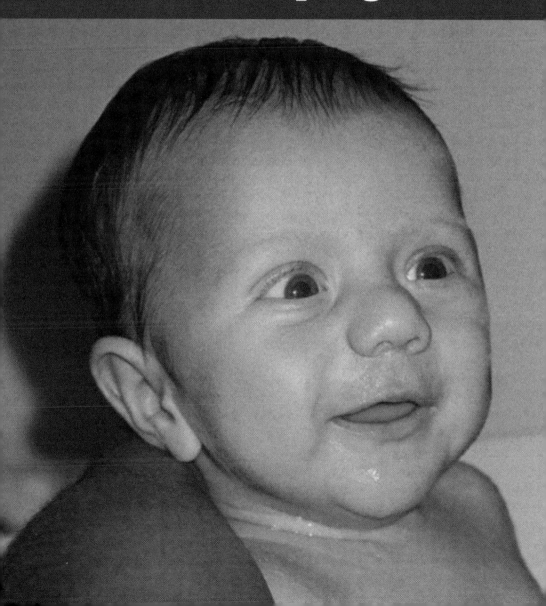

Chapter 2

Trying to get pregnant

> I had waited until I became a consultant; there was no way I could have had children as a medical registrar, but then it was eight years before I got pregnant.
>
> *Consultant physician*

Having spent the best part of your life trying not to get pregnant, it can be more than a bit frustrating if you now find that you can't. Despite being medics, you may not have thought about gynaecology for many years, so it might help to swat up on the advice recommended by the Royal College of Obstetricians and Gynaecologists (NICE recommendations). If you have regular sex (classed as every 2–3 days) without contraception, about 84 of every 100 couples will get pregnant within a year. About 92 of every 100 couples will get pregnant in 2 years.

For women aged 35, 94% will get pregnant within 3 years of trying. For women aged 38, 77% will get pregnant.

1. Have sex every 2–3 days throughout the month, not just when you think you may be most fertile.
2. A body mass index (BMI) of less than 19 or more than 29 may reduce your chances of getting pregnant.
3. Stopping smoking may improve your fertility.
4. Avoid drinking more than one or two units of alcohol once or twice a week to avoid the possibility of harming a developing embryo. Recent advice from the Department of Health advocating abstinence is not based on any new evidence or findings.
5. There is no consistent evidence of a link between caffeine intake and fertility problems.

Take 0.4 mg of folic acid daily for 3 months before you start trying, and for the first 3 months of the pregnancy.

If you are taking medication for epilepsy, or have previously had a baby with spina bifida, you may be advised to take 5 mg of folic acid daily.

> I'd planned to try and get pregnant at some point during my two year rotation, thinking that it took most women at least a year or so ... All you ever hear about is women trying for ages ... Then I got pregnant the first time we tried, and it completely threw us, I ended up having a baby right at the start of my training.
>
> *ST medicine*

Your mother may advise you that eating three regular meals a day, getting 8 hours sleep a night, and doing a headstand after sex are all useful. Unless she is a doctor, she won't understand that you don't have time to eat (or the canteen only serves food when you're on a ward round or in theatre), you never get 8 hours of sleep a night (because life's too short), and when you manage to summon up the energy to have sex you'd rather fall asleep afterwards than do yoga.

Working while undergoing IVF

As a woman undergoing in-vitro fertilization (IVF), you may be classed as a Category 1 applicant for flexible training (see Chapter 12).

How to calculate your estimated delivery date (EDD)

A pregnancy lasts, on average, 280 days (40 weeks). Day 1 is the first day of your last menstrual period. To calculate your EDD, simply:

1. Determine the first day of your last period.
2. Count back three calendar months from that date.
3. Add 1 year and 7 days to that date.

The above three stages are Naegele's Rule, and are based on a 28-day cycle. You need to adjust the dates for longer or shorter cycles. If your cycle is longer than 28 days, for example, 31 days, then add 3 days to your EDD. If your cycle is shorter, for example, is 26 days, then subtract 2 days from the EDD. Once you have done all your sums, you need to bear in mind that not only is Naegele's rule apparently rather unreliable, but that only about 10% of babies come on their due dates. Maybe it's because we all have to make wild guesses as to the date of our last period to the midwife, because we were too busy working/dealing with small children/internet shopping to write it down in the Filofax.

If your brain can't cope after a long day at work, then you can access online calendars for estimating your EDD, such as the one at http://www.emmasdiary.co.uk, or search Google for 'EDD calculator.'

Foods you are advised to avoid by NICE once you find out you're pregnant

(Your patients will be horrified if they spot you scoffing a nut-encrusted foie gras and camembert sandwich between surgeries.)

- Mould-ripened soft cheeses such as camembert, Brie, and blue-veined cheeses
- Unpasteurized milk
- Raw shellfish

- Raw eggs
- Pate
- Raw or undercooked meat, especially poultry
- Liver, and supplements containing vitamin A

References

NICE Guidelines (October 2003) *Antenatal Care. Routine care for the healthy pregnant woman*. Clinical Guideline 6.

NICE Guidelines (February 2004) Understanding NICE guidelines—information for people with fertility problems, their partners, and the public. *Fertility: Assessment and treatment for people with fertility problems.* Reference number NO466.

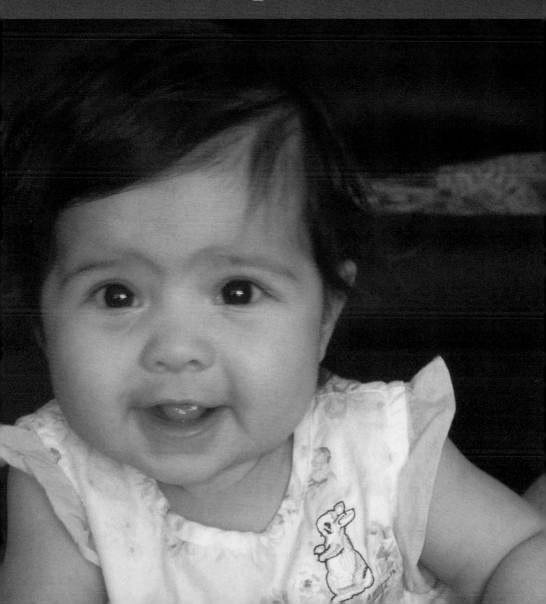

Chapter 3

Life as a pregnant hospital doctor

You do manage it, but sometimes that's hard to believe, particularly with your first child … Some people bounce through pregnancy like a spring rabbit, but I just lay on the sofa and gestated for nine months … I was the world's worst pregnant woman… I even got the nickname of El Nino … Whenever I did an operation, it went wrong, a disaster occurred!

Consultant surgeon

You may discover that you're pregnant quite early on, or you may find that several weeks or even months have passed before you realize that something is not quite right. My mum informed me that I was pregnant when my embryo was the size of a spec of dust, because I told her I was 'tired all the time,' (a GP's worst nightmare?) Not bad for a spot diagnosis down the telephone, although I still had to buy two pregnancy testing kits (that's four tests) just to check, plus another test about 2 months later, just to check. I have to say that the joys of doing a pregnancy test when you actually want to be pregnant are immeasurable, but try to avoid the temptation of taking a test at work and doing it in the staff loo, because you'll probably cry and have red eyes for the rest of the day.

> As soon as you know you are pregnant, make an appointment with occupational health, even if you don't want to tell anyone else at work yet. They can advise you on what you need to do, and when.

I had to tell someone as soon as I knew I was pregnant; I told the person who was co-coordinating the rota, another reg … I couldn't do certain things on call. There were lots of trauma calls though, and you just had to do it … You double gown [with lead] and just get on with it, try and stand as far back as you can, stuff like that. We had a junior and a senior on call, and if I couldn't do it, like a screening procedure, I couldn't do it. By eight or nine weeks, everyone at work knew [that I was pregnant] … Before my family, in fact!

ST radiology

The problem with finding out so soon is that you then have to endure about 2 months of worrying about a miscarriage before you start to relax. If you're too busy filling out your assessment forms/going to meetings/trying to stay awake after nights, and a while passes before you realize you haven't had a period, at least you've already clocked off some of the 40 weeks. You may then spend a while wondering how many times you've been mid-catheter when someone announced, from beyond the curtain, that they were taking a portable chest X-ray.

My friend [another registrar] had to tell the people where we were working [that she was pregnant] … It was the first time that a female trainee had done anything so radical, in what was then a very male dominated speciality ... Then not long after, I got pregnant, and we were under pressure with the rota, we were short staffed. I hadn't told anyone, but in fact I was feeling grotty and extremely tired, and the consultant said to me 'Look, why is it that you don't want to do more?' I said 'Well actually, I'm pregnant; it's very early, and I haven't told anyone yet, not even my family, so I don't want to take on extra work.' He was a bit shocked, as I was the second female in such a short time, and he was quite old school. Then about two weeks later, a friend of mine, who was the secretary for another consultant in another hospital I'd worked at, she rang me up and said 'Congratulations!' I asked her how on earth she knew, and it turned out that my consultant had told her consultant, and actually quite a few people, some of whom knew my parents, had been told ... I was really angry, and then I thought well, I'd better tell my parents!

Consultant nephrologist

First trimester

How you cope at work is very dependent on the job you are doing at the time, your grade, and the support of your team. It also depends, of course, on your health and on any pregnancy-related problems you may have. I was a junior house officer in surgery (FY1) during the first part of my pregnancy, which in my books was about as bad as it could get, but I was very lucky to have a fabulously supportive consultant. He bent over backwards for me, and did everything he could to make sure I was OK.

In clinic, she [the SHO] had morning sickness, and was vomiting in between patients ... She never took a day off sick ... There was this great bravado about her, her consultant thought she was just marvellous.

ST dermatology

If you have a miscarriage (classed as before the 25th week of pregnancy) you are entitled to normal sick leave, even if you think you should be back at work the next day. If you have a threatened miscarriage, talking to your bosses may reveal them to be more sympathetic than you think, and you are entitled to time off.

I was on call, and on my way to theatre ... I felt a bit uncomfortable, so I went to the loo, and realised [that I was having a miscarriage] ... I didn't know what it was going to be like, so I just got on with the operation... But within the hour, oh my god, eventually I just keeled over in the corner. Nobody knew [that I was pregnant] ... I remember coming round, with the anaesthetist trying to resuscitate me, with my boss shouting his head off at me, I heard '... And how the **** am I supposed to operate if the ******* assistant is on the ******* floor!' The female anaesthetist hauled me into the female changing room, and I explained what was happening, then she started prescribing all sorts of stuff. She jabbed something into my thigh, voltarol I suppose, then he [my boss] came in and shouted 'What the hell was all that about?!' and the anaesthetist just shouted at him 'She's having a miscarriage, you unfeeling giant!' He was really taken aback, he felt terrible, and I could hear him through the toilet door, saying how awful he felt ...

Consultant surgeon

I came out from the scan [after having a miscarriage], and walked straight into one of the consultants ... He knew what had happened; it had gone round the department ... He took one look at me, and said 'Come here, love,' and gave me a huge hug. He was such a crusty old gentleman, I never thought he'd be like that, but he was just wonderful.

Consultant surgeon

Who you should tell at work, and when

The laws that protect you at work when you are pregnant only apply once your employer knows (i.e. is given written notice) that you are pregnant.

By the 15th week before your baby is due (when you are about 25 weeks pregnant)

- Tell your employer, in writing, that you're pregnant
- Tell them when you want your maternity leave and maternity pay to start
- Your maternity leave can start any time from 11 weeks before the baby is due (when you are about 29 weeks pregnant)
- Give your employer the Mat B1 form from your GP or midwife (take a photocopy first!)
- Your partner must tell their employer at this time that they want to take paternity leave, or they could in theory be denied it if they leave it until later (See the standard form SC3 on the website www.directgov.uk/employees).

You can change your mind about when you want to start your maternity leave, but you are supposed to give 28 days notice of the change.

If you aren't planning to take the full maternity leave, you need to let your employer know when you'll be coming back—you can change your mind later on, but you should give 8 weeks notice of the change.

If you change your mind and want to come back later, you should make sure you give 8 weeks notice before the original (earlier) date.

Advice from the Health and Safety Executive (HSE)

It's difficult [planning pregnancy] in radiology ... There are certain lists you can't do once you're pregnant, and where I work we do blocks ... So you do a block of CT, or a block of ultrasound, for three months at a time ... If you were doing something like interventional radiology, and you got pregnant, you'd have to change blocks.

ST radiology

Once you notify your employer that you are pregnant, they have to carry out a risk assessment of the work you do. Below is a list of risks, identified by the HSE, which should be avoided if possible. (See Chapter 7 for more detailed information.)

- Lifting/carrying of heavy loads
- Standing or sitting for long lengths of time
- Exposure to infectious disease
- Exposure to lead
- Work-related stress
- Workstations and posture
- Exposure to radioactive material
- Other people's smoke in the workplace
- Threat of violence in the workplace
- Long working hours
- Excessively noisy workplaces

In order to avoid the risks outlined above, most doctors would have to leave work. As doctors, most of us have had to fight bigger battles than simply being pregnant at work, and very few would take the rules above too literally; otherwise, we couldn't do our jobs, which we have been trained to do, and which (most of the time) we love. The key is in finding a balance that allows you to continue being a doctor, in a job that interests you, while looking after yourself and your baby. You may have moments of sheer madness when you forget to be careful, and I almost injected myself with testosterone during a urology clinic, but in general we're a sensible bunch of people.

When I was a house officer there was another house officer who was pregnant for about half the year ... They really looked after her ... We were doing orthopaedics, it was a really quiet job for us, and they didn't make her go to theatre if she didn't want to ...

GP

A girl at X Hospital, a Registrar, she was pregnant and having loads of problems with sickness and tiredness and everything, and she couldn't do her on-calls ... And it causes loads of tension, because, well you're not capable of doing the job, and people resent you for that.

ST surgery

The following actions are supposed to be monitored and reviewed on a regular basis, once you have notified your employer, in writing, that you are pregnant (see Chapter 7 for more information).

1. Carry out a risk assessment that is specific to you, to take into account any medical advice from your GP or midwife.
2. If a risk is identified, can the risk be removed?
3. If the risk cannot be removed, can your working hours/working conditions be adjusted (at the same rate of pay)?
4. If not, can you be given suitable alternative work on the same terms and conditions (i.e. at the same rate of pay)?
5. If you cannot be given suitable alternative work, you must be suspended from work, on fully paid leave, for as long as is necessary to protect your health and safety, or that of your child.

Remember that if you are on a rotation and changing jobs during pregnancy, you'll need to have a new risk assessment carried out for each job.

My partner, she's a radiology registrar, and when she was pregnant they found her lots of work she could do sitting down... Reporting and stuff... So she didn't get too tired.

ST medicine

There were no guidelines in place as to what a heavily pregnant woman should do, with on calls and that ... It's a case by case set up, rather than actual guidelines being in place.

ST medicine

At about 30 weeks I started to get hypertension and proteinuria, so they pulled me out of on calls ... The GP said so, so I went to occupational health ... They said 'Right, do you want us to tell him [your boss] or you? Who do you work for?' When they saw who it was, they said 'Oh no ...' But I wanted it to come from them so it would be official, I didn't want to be the soft woman who can't pull her weight at work.

Consultant surgeon

You should have realized by now that my mum is a wise lady and a great friend to me. I had made the decision, once I found out that I was pregnant, not to tell anyone

Tips on being a hospital doctor during the first trimester

- If you don't normally carry a bag, get one! A bottle of water (which you can refill), and snacks, will be very welcome during the post-take ward round/clinic. You can feel incredibly thirsty during the early days, and savoury snacks can help stave off nausea.

- Keep your ears open for portable X-rays if you're on the wards/in resus (it might sound obvious, but some radiographers shout very quietly).

- Needle sticks are never a good idea, especially now; don't take unnecessary risks, and if you do get one, make sure you get advice from the virologist on call (not the occupational health answering machine).

- If you are unlucky enough to develop a sense of smell like a bloodhound, practise mouth breathing.

- If you are suffering from devastating tiredness, remember that it will pass (normally by about 12 weeks). Try getting one or two really, really early nights.

in my team. My mum had other ideas, and advised me to confide in a female member of my team, not necessarily a doctor, but someone with whom I worked closely. She said it would make an enormous difference in the early days, and she was right. Whether it was a kind cup of tea slipped under my nose when I least expected it, or someone to share a smile with every morning, it really helped to know that someone else knew my amazing news. After a while you may end up blurting it out to everyone anyway, because it's just so exciting and you can't resist it, and that definitely helps explain some of your weird behaviour (some annoying people will have realized that you're pregnant anyway, reminding you that you didn't drink anything at the mess party or that you've been looking a bit peaky).

> When I was pregnant, and having problems, I didn't tell other doctors... They just know the scary stuff. I talked to other mums, who were generally full of good common sense advice!
>
> *ST general practice*

Telling your team will help if you've been suffering with extreme tiredness, morning sickness, or a bladder which needs to empty every 5 minutes. I have a memory of leaving two male consultants, one male registrar, one male SHO and two male medical students, standing in the corridor outside the ladies loo in the middle of a ward round, looking like a bunch of naughty boys at school. They were very sweet about it, but I was mortified. If you are a consultant, sharing your news may be a breath of fresh air to your juniors, who can now stop thinking they were the cause of your problems.

Second trimester

> I had to have a bit of time off at about 13 weeks, because I fell down the stairs and hurt my back … I felt really guilty being off work … Like it was an excuse.
>
> *Consultant physician*

For many women, this time is the best bit. Suddenly, you have a 'bump', and everyone will be saying 'Ooh, you're having a baby!', as if you didn't know already (apart from the occasional doctor, who will be surprised to hear your news, despite the fact that you're carrying a watermelon). If you're really lucky, you might even get offered a seat on the bus to work. Now is also the time to start thinking about maternity clothes, which can strike the fear of god into your heart at first, but which really aren't that bad. Squeezing yourself into your normal work clothes for as long as possible will only mean that your tops will look too short and your waistline will become ischaemic. There can be a slightly disturbing time when you don't look pregnant, but you're not the woman you once were, and you end feeling like you've eaten all the pies. You may even wonder if the baby is growing in the cheeks of your bottom. It is worth spending a bit of money on a few basic bits and pieces, such as black trousers and a few tops, then you can supplement them with cheaper tops from maternity ranges at high street shops, such as Top Shop and Dorothy Perkins. You buy your normal size, but in the maternity range; some will also have different 'stages', such as 'size 12, 6–9 months.' The reason for buying a few nice pieces is that you will end up wearing these things day in, day out, for some time. If you find something you like, buy two. It's probably worth thinking about footwear at this point too, as one day in a pair of nice heels may lead to swollen ankles for a week.

Online shopping sites for maternity clothes

www.bloomingmarvellous.co.uk

www.bumpsmaternity.com

www.bump2babe.co.uk

www.dorothyperkins.co.uk

www.fromheretomaternity.co.uk

www.isabellaoliver.com

www.jojomamanbebe.co.uk/

www.mamasandpapas.co.uk

www.melbaclothing.com

www.maternityexchange.co.uk

www.mindthebump.co.uk

www.next.co.uk

www.picchumaternity.com

www.seraphine.com

www.topshop.com

I was in training to do obs and gynae before I had children. I was working in an IVF department when I was pregnant, and as soon as I started to show, they put me out the back doing stuff other than seeing patients … It was a bit weird, but I suppose I could see why.

ST medicine

During the second trimester of my pregnancy (as a surgical PRHO on a vascular firm), I was fortunate enough to have an SHO from heaven. Not only did she support me both physically and emotionally, she was kind enough to have a phantom pregnancy with all the signs and symptoms I managed to personally avoid; nausea in the mornings, bloating, and even swollen ankles. The support you get from your team can be the difference between a happy pregnancy and a miserable one.

I was having a lot of back pain, and when we were on call we had to set up the filter machines ourselves in intensive care, which were quite heavy … So I stopped my on calls then [at about 24 weeks].

Consultant nephrologist

Changing jobs during pregnancy

- Don't apologize for being pregnant when you arrive on your first day!
- Inform your new boss before you arrive unless you have fairly thick skin
- Make sure you have notified your new employer and HR of your intended date for going on maternity leave
- If you are also moving house, make sure you register with a new GP as soon as possible, and find out about local maternity services; you'll need to book with the local hospital unless you're having a home birth
- Go to occupational health at your new hospital as soon as possible
- Check with HR at your new hospital that they have a copy of your Mat B1 certificate
- Try and get hold of a copy of the rota as soon as possible

I did an interdeanery transfer in the middle of my pregnancy, as well as my exams, because my husband had got a job up here … I thought oh god, they've given me the job I wanted, and they've been so great about it, and they've taken me on a transfer, and now I've gone and buggered it up and I'm going to have to tell them I'm pregnant, and I want to come back part time, and I don't even know them....

And they're surgeons! But they were absolutely delightful, they were fantastic.

Consultant surgeon

You will also need some time off for antenatal appointments; you are entitled to paid time off to attend these, and despite the temptation to dip your own urine or do your own scan, it's best to go. Having said that, you might find that arranging your appointments in the hospital you work at is easiest. 'Self-scanning' is not recommended; if you think you can see horns, or a tail, you'll just panic and end up taking more time off to go to a proper appointment anyway. You'll know in advance when you need to be at the hospital or doctor's surgery, so at least you can warn your team and plan things a bit.

Quite early on [at my ante-natal appointments], when I had high blood pressure and oedema, people gave me the choice [because they knew I was a doctor], they would say 'Well what do you want to do,' and I would think, look just do what you have to, just because I'm a doctor, don't give me the choice!

Consultant renal physician

You can arrange to have all your antenatal appointments at the hospital you're working at … Some people might find that a bit weird, but in the long run it's much easier, as you don't need to take half a day off every time you've got a check-up.

ST paediatrics

Rough schedule of antenatal appointments

- Booking appointment (about 12 weeks); this is your first antenatal appointment after you discover that you're pregnant. Allow at least half an hour, as the midwife will need lots of information. You'll be given an appointment for a dating scan, to confirm your due date. Nuchal translucency is usually done at the same time as the dating scan.
- The frequency of antenatal visits will depend on your health, and on the number of children you've had. A rough guide is that you are seen monthly from booking up to 26 weeks, then fortnightly until 36 weeks, then weekly until delivery.
- Remember that if you're Rhesus negative you'll need a couple of extra appointments for your anti-D injections.

If you need amniocentesis, it usually happens between 15 and 18 weeks.

A long time since medical school? How to interpret your maternity records if you are a dermatologist:

- FHH—Fetal heart heard
- FMF—Fetal movement felt
- Cx—Cervix
- Vx—Vertex presentation; well flexed head, the ideal attitude (degree of flexion)
- OT—occipito-transverse (position of the head, to describe its rotation—OP is occipito-posterior, OA is occipito-anterior)
- Fundal height—The distance from the pubic bone to the fundus
- Relation of PP to Brim—The position of the baby's presenting part (head or bottom) with relation to the brim of the pelvis

Impey, L. (1999) *Obstetrics and gynaecology*. Blackwell Publishing, Oxford

Third trimester

You may start feeling tired again, or you may feel fine right until the end. Some women have problems with their back, constipation, piles and a bladder that keeps them on the move, while others just sail through. I found myself increasingly wary of drunk, violent customers in A&E, and it's probably just best to steer clear. Your baby will be dancing along to the relentless sound of your bleep going off in its ear every 5 seconds, and may enjoy pushing you away from the desk as you try and type at the computer, or bouncing your clip board up and down in meetings.

The main issue for hospital doctors in the final part of pregnancy can be mobility, or lack of it. Towards the end, all activities that involve fast movement become more difficult, and you may find that you don't have to carry the crash bleep. There are laws in place to protect you, and it's difficult not to try and keep up with your colleagues, but you might need to take it easy at times. You may still want to do your on-calls, which will differ depending on what grade you are in, and what job you are doing.

> I consciously chose not to have a baby until I was a consultant … I wouldn't have thought of it as a registrar. My pregnancy was fine; I worked until a few days before the end. Being a [pregnant] consultant on call, I mean it's coming in on weekends and that, but it's nothing like having to do nights on the ward… It's much easier as a consultant.
>
> *Consultant geriatrician*

Surviving nights during late pregnancy

You may be doing nights in terms of being up all night covering the wards and A&E, or you may be in a job that allows you to go to bed and rest in between calls from the ward. If you're up and working all night, the following may be helpful:

- It sounds obvious but make sure you try and rest in the day. If you have other children at home to look after, try and arrange childcare for that day, or at least for a few hours in the afternoon. Try and arrange childcare for the following morning too.
- Take plenty of food and drink with you for the night as there may not be anywhere to buy it; then make sure you eat it.

If you're lucky enough to be able to go to bed for a while:

- If you can, take in your own pillows or cushions; by now you may find it very hard to get comfortable, and there's nothing worse than finding that the on-call room has an uncomfortable bed. You may find it helpful to put a thin pillow under your 'bump' as you now have to sleep on your side.
- If you're having problems with back ache, make sure you either take in a hot water bottle, or try and borrow a heat pad from one of the wards.
- Doing a late ward round and troubleshooting, however exhausted you feel in the late evening, may mean that you get a few hours without interruptions. Tell all the nurses in charge when you will be doing another round, say at 6 a.m., and some things may be able to wait until then.

Working late (evenings)

If you are a junior doctor working a late shift, and working all day too, you may find that you can try and get 10 minutes rest or so before you come 'on call.' If you're working all day, then come 'on call' at 5 p.m., you shouldn't (in theory) get too many calls around 5 p.m., except for handovers for jobs to be done later. Try asking your team if you can disappear at quarter to five while someone else holds the bleep, to try and get a few minutes rest before the evening. You might be able to find a quiet office, but if your library is not too far away, that's often a great place to get a few minutes peace and quiet! Remember that most people will be very understanding of your situation.

Remember not to feel guilty if you are struggling. You may find that just winding back a bit one week is all you need, and you can be back on form the next week. The priority is to look after yourself and the baby.

I was carrying twins, and I carried on until 35 weeks, it was fine.

ST paediatrics

All it is, it's an adjustment, and it's a temporary state …

Consultant surgeon

Doing exams when you're pregnant

Tell the college that you're pregnant, as they may be able to make things easier for you, such as sitting you near the door by the toilets! Also, remember not to leave it to the last minute to find something smart to wear; your suit may not fit you anymore.

I had my first attempt [at exit exams] at 28 weeks, which was a disaster, and again at 38 and a half weeks … But because I was so full of happy hormones, I couldn't have given a monkeys if I passed or not … I took my husband with me, in case I went into labour … And in fact the college was brilliant… There was a choice of two hospitals [to sit the exam at], and they booked me into the one which had maternity facilities … The written bit was in a lecture theatre, and they put me in a desk at the front, because I couldn't physically sit behind the desks [in the lecture theatre] … They checked the ladies toilet just outside the door, that there were no books in it, and they said 'Look, if your bladder's full and you've got to go, just go!' The only problems I had doing the exam were physical problems … The chaps were being very non touchy feely, but I needed a crane to get up and down off the floor, and they gave me feet to examine! The final straw was the long case patient, who was a lovely lady with multiple joint pathologies, she was practically crippled, I was in a hopeless state too, and we both just ended up in hysterical laughter… She couldn't move, and I couldn't help her!

Consultant orthopaedic surgeon

I did MRCPath about a month before I gave birth … I was completely nonchalant about the whole thing because I just felt like a whale, I was so exhausted … But I passed! It just goes to show … Being more laid-back probably got me through the exam.

ST haematology

Swollen ankles

Aside from pathological causes, you may find that spending hours on your feet or hours sitting still in clinics makes your ankles swell. If you have to spend long periods of time standing still in theatre, try and get hold of some TED (antithrombotic) stockings. If you have a friendly tissue viability nurse, they may be able to advise you on some hosiery that stops it happening. Remember not to wear TEDS if you're going out in a skirt that night; you'll have lovely red ridges on display.

As a consultant, it was much easier; I was much more sure of my life, and it's much easier to be assertive about these things when you're the boss... I worried about being on call, and having a registrar struggle with a nail ... So I talked to a few other consultants, and they said don't worry, just call us ... But that was terrifying, much worse than having to ring the boss at night when you're a reg, but in fact I never needed to call them!

Consultant orthopaedic surgeon

If you need time off sick, or have to be admitted to hospital during the pregnancy

If you are unwell with an illness not related to pregnancy, your normal sickness pay rules apply up to the date that you've notified for the start of your maternity leave.

If your illness is related to pregnancy, and you're ill after the fourth week before the expected week of childbirth (about 36 weeks onwards) SMP or MA will start from the first day after you are absent from work (see Chapter 8).

Occasional days of pregnancy related illness can apparently be taken as normal sick days at the discretion of the employer.

I stopped work at thirty seven and a half weeks ... It's quite good, radiology, in terms of sitting down, and you could always have a glass of water with you, things like that made it easier.

ST radiology

You are entitled to time off for antenatal classes, although you will know well in advance when these are going to be, so you can plan accordingly. Don't think that because you're a doctor you know it all; do you know how to latch a baby on to breastfeed? Were you really listening in the obs and gynae lectures all those years ago anyway? They can seem a bit tedious at times, but whatever you do don't let on that you're a doctor, or it will be assumed that you've delivered hundreds of babies and you know everything. Most classes include a tour of the antenatal unit, which is very useful (unless you're having a home birth).

Attitudes of other staff

People will look at you differently, depending on the grade you're working in, and depending on whether they themselves have had children. Some people believe that pregnancy is a normal state, and that you can carry on as usual. Others may appear horrified that you're running with the crash bleep at 24 weeks gestation. Most staff and patients will be very positive about the fact that you're pregnant. If you're a senior registrar, or a consultant, your junior female staff will be looking up to you as a role model. I was told off by a nurse for running on the ward when I was 7 weeks pregnant; she was worried about me falling over. She had no idea that I would ice skate, as I have done since the age of 5, until I was 6 months pregnant. Another nurse (a male nurse, from Germany,) was appalled that I was working while pregnant. He said that back home, I wouldn't be allowed, because of all the risks. Each time you encounter attitudes like this, you just have to grin and bear it; it's your life, and your pregnancy. All over the world, women work until late into their pregnancies.

Many doctors try and work as late as possible into the pregnancy, in order to have plenty of time off afterwards with the baby. If you can only afford to take 3 months off, then you may feel pressured if you're exhausted near the end (see Chapter 8). When I was 6 months pregnant, I had no idea how I would feel by 36 weeks. I was clearly struggling at the very end, evidenced by the fact that I spent every morning handover lying on the floor with my legs in the air, trying to regain consciousness, but I know that many women successfully work until just days before they give birth. Like everything else to do with pregnancy and motherhood, you have to do what feels right for you and not try and be superwoman.

> I had a bit of a problem with blood pressure ... I did the on-calls, the days, until about 36 weeks [as a medical registrar] but they were shifts by then, and if you did a day on call, you didn't have to do the night too ... I stopped my nights at about 30 weeks. I had oedema and high blood pressure. There were two other pregnant registrars, so it was all a bit awkward.
>
> Consultant physician

Remember—you do not have to decide how much maternity leave you want to take yet, so don't get stressed about it during pregnancy or in the early precious days with your baby. Obviously, it helps to give your employer a rough idea, but with enough notice (8 weeks) you can change your mind.

On your final day at work, you may feel a little strange. After all, can you imagine having a whole year off work? The last few days can be stressful, as you need to sort out proper handovers and tie up all the lose ends, but bear in mind that soon, you will have a few days or weeks to put your feet up and rest (unless you've left all your baby shopping to the last minute).

References

Department of Trade and Industry (2007) *Pregnancy and Work: What you need to know as an employer. Babies due on or after 1 April 2007*. Department of Trade and Industry, London.

Chapter 4

Life as a pregnant general practitioner

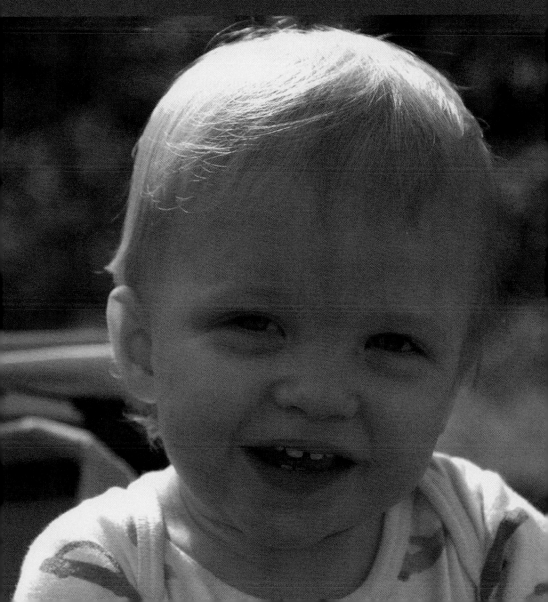

The minute it was noticeable that I was pregnant, my relationship with my patients changed, definitely for the better. In general practice, I guess you find out so much about other people, they're desperate to know a little bit about you ... And then suddenly there's this very obvious thing about you, on show ... And they have this lovely sort of 'ownership' of the baby ... Even now, I would say in about half of my consultations, the patient will walk in and say 'How's the baby?' And it's lovely ... They feel like they know me a little bit better... And because I've shared a little bit of me, maybe not consciously, I've got a better relationship with them. For me, that's just been so positive.

GP

Depending on the speciality you work in, you may think that GPs have it easy when it comes to pregnancy. There are no long ward rounds, no crash calls to the fifth floor, and no standing in theatre for hours on end. Most people would agree that general practice is a very family friendly occupation, and that GPs are in general supportive of their pregnant colleagues.

[My partner] brought in a duvet and a pillow for me so I could have a nap in-between surgeries ... He couldn't have been nicer!

GP

There are, of course, pitfalls to working in general practice during pregnancy, namely the continuous stream of patients with coughs of colds, and children with strange looking rashes. Once you've called your mum in a panic to check that you definitely, absolutely did have chicken pox when you were a child, you might be able to relax a bit, but it might feel as if the world and his dog are out to infect you and your baby with something, even if it's just the popular virus of the moment.

So when you're 13 weeks pregnant, and nobody at work knows, and someone walks in with their two kids and says 'They've got chicken pox' ... You end up feeling really stressed, thinking, why did you bring them in here then?!

GP

The only hassle with general practice is ... You have exposure to lots of illnesses all the time ... I remember seeing one guy [when I was pregnant], well in the end he had septic shock; he came in with a purpuric rash, and I saw it, as soon as he walked in to my room, I sat him down, moved to the phone, and called an ambulance... He crashed in the ambulance on the way to hospital ... My only thought was, well I don't know if I'm going to have to take prophylaxis ... Or whether I can... I just wanted to get him out of my room as soon as possible, yet that was what saved his life probably!

GP

Unlike hospital consultants, GP partners are effectively in charge of a small business. Many GPs feel guilty about going on maternity leave, and leaving their partners to 'run the show' without them, as well as having to find extra money to cover the cost of a locum. It might be difficult deciding when to tell your partners that you are about to take 6 months off with full pay, despite knowing that the PCT won't cover the costs, but as with all things pregnancy-related, sooner is usually better than later.

I felt very supported [by my partners], but there's a constant guilt feeling with going away ... It must be the same for lots of GP's ... Because you're part of a small business, and the effects that [going on maternity leave] will have... I'm sure it will be fine, but it's quite stressful really. Ultimately most GPs will be part of a family, and even the men have wives who've had to do it... So they understand.

GP

[One of the Partners] is on the LMC [Local Medical Committee], and he's been in negotiations with the PCT about how much reimbursement we get... £1200 a week I think, which is really good ... I get six months full pay... But I know in other areas it's not like that. But my friend, in [another area], she's becoming a partner and negotiating her maternity pay, and there are a lot of older women partners, who are saying 'Well when we did it, we had to take holiday, and miss out on our pensions, and we don't think you should get it ...' she's actually getting 3 months full pay, and 3 months half pay ... Another one, she's a partner, and until she's been a partner for two years she'd have to pay for a locum herself ... Some GPs are doing ok and can afford that, but no way... That'd be crippling.

GP

For GMS practices (General Medical Services,) where a partnership employs a locum in order to cover a colleague who is away on maternity leave, they will be entitled to claim an amount of money from the PCT, towards the cost of that locum. The period of time which that payment is to cover has been increased to 26 weeks, in line with the statutory provision for employees. PMS practices (Personal Medical Services) have to reach an agreement with their primary care organization.

I told the other partners when I was about 15 weeks pregnant... I was absolutely dreading it. I decided to tell X, who I knew would be the more difficult one ... They knew I'd had some time off, been to some 'appointments', I'd been for the scan and stuff… He came in, and he said 'Is everything ok?' and I said 'Yes, everything's fine, except that I'm pregnant.' And he said 'Oh, sh**!' And then there was some silence for a bit. And then he said 'Well, that's very good news. For you.' So we exchanged a few polite words, then I left the room.

GP

As a registrar in general practice, despite the fact that you are employed by the practice rather than the NHS, there has been a long-standing agreement with the health department that GP registrars are entitled to the same maternity pay and leave as hospital doctors. Ultimately, it depends on your practice. See Chapter 8 for more information.

Salaried GPs should find their maternity rights described in their individual contracts.

GP principles are, as a result of their self-employed status, not covered by the NHS maternity scheme. Your contract will tell you what maternity leave and pay you are entitled to.

Maternity leave and pay for partners in general practice will be laid out in their individual contract.

(For further details on GP maternity leave go to Chapter 8.)

The registrar year is a really great time to be pregnant … I planned my first baby for that time … It's a good year to go for it, even though you've got your [assessments] and things.

GP

Patients generally love the fact that you're pregnant. You'll be referred to as 'the pregnant doctor' if they can't remember your name, and like pregnant hospital doctors, your patients may even feel sorry for you when work is hectic. All pregnant doctors, wherever they work, may wish they had a badge, stating 'Yes, I am pregnant. The baby is due on XXX. I don't know if it's a boy or a girl. It's my first baby. Yes, I am quite tired.' Perhaps there could be Quality Outcome Framework points awarded if all queries about the baby are answered and you still manage to get the patient out of the door within 7 minutes.

In the last month, people have started noticing … Initially I found it a bit intrusive, because you don't ask personal questions about anything else … To begin with they didn't say much, but now, a lot of people ask whether it's a girl, when your due date is, but sometimes, it can actually be really distracting … In some ways, it's really nice, especially in antenatal clinic, but also, when you're seeing older

[Bengali] women, with a translator, and all they're doing is translating questions about your baby, it's really hard to get them back on track, and get everything done in ten minutes!

ST general practice

Who you should tell at work, and when
Advice from the Health and Safety Executive

Once you notify your employer that you are pregnant, they have to carry out a risk assessment of the work you do. Below is a list if risks, identified by the HSE, which should be avoided if possible. (See Chapter 7 for more detailed information.)

- Lifting/carrying of heavy loads
- Standing or sitting for long lengths of time
- Exposure to infectious disease
- Exposure to lead
- Work-related stress
- Workstations and posture
- Exposure to radioactive material
- Other people's smoke in the workplace
- Threat of violence in the workplace
- Long working hours
- Excessively noisy workplaces

The main advantage you have over your colleagues in the hospital is that you no longer have to do nights on call, running around the corridors with the crash bleep, or standing for hours on post-take ward rounds. Your Out of Hours (OOH) should be fairly civilized, but if you're suffering, talk to one of your partners for help.

Generally, it was ok, but home visits were a struggle when I was eight months pregnant, you'd get to a block of flats and the lift was broken, you'd have to struggle up with your doctor's bag …

GP

The GP Returner Scheme
....

The scheme was developed to help doctors who had been off work for more than 2 years to return to work in general practice. The government withdrew central funding in early 2006, and since then the scheme has virtually disappeared, despite helping about 550 GPs return to the NHS in 4 years. See the Royal College of General Practitioners website for the latest updates.

- www.rcgp.org.uk

As a GP, you'll have dealt with numerous pregnant women; you probably did at least one job in obstetrics, and you may do the antenatal clinic every week. For those reasons, it can be quite tempting to do your own antenatal appointments. After all, one of your colleagues can stick you with anti-D, and you can play 'listen to the baby's heartbeat' in between consultations. It must be very frustrating, when you know what you're talking about, to spend hours travelling to and from antenatal appointments, waiting around, taking time off work, only to be told what you already knew (or to be told things that you know are complete rubbish). Is there anything worse than being sent to an antenatal appointment at the hospital, only to be seen by the new FY2 in obstetrics, on day 3 of their job?

> My current debate is whether to disclose if you're a health professional … To your midwife or whatever … And I've tried to be a good patient, and go to my appointments, and take my advice … But actually I've had really **** advice … This morning, I went to my antenatal appointment, and I was measuring below the week by 1 cm … And I know the protocol, it's scan if its below 3 cm … And I was told 'Look, it's really small … Are you still working?' And 'Right, once you stop work, you must put your feet up, and drink lots of milk …' I mean what the hell is all that about? Is drinking lots of milk based on any evidence?! [One of the partners] thinks it's unfair of me to just take this, without questioning it … And I think it's difficult, there's so much clap trap and old wives tales… It is really irritating to get advice like that.
>
> *GP*

GPs as employers

Unlike hospital consultants, whose colleagues are employed by the NHS, GP partners are self-employed, and employ other staff, such as salaried GPs.

As soon as your employee tells you she is pregnant

- You need to carry out a risk assessment, and make necessary alternative arrangements.
- You must allow them to have paid time off for ante-natal appointments.
- You can then plan for her leave.
- Does she have any annual leave to take before her maternity leave starts?
- Make arrangements to cover her leave.
- If she is off sick with a pregnancy-related problem you have to pay her in the same way as for any other illness.

Within 28 days of receiving your employee's dates for maternity leave

- You are obliged to write to your employee, telling her when she is due back at work.

- Tell her if she can get Statutory Maternity Pay (SMP), and how much (she will qualify for SMP if she has been employed by you continuously for 26 weeks by 15 weeks before the week her baby is due).
- If she doesn't qualify for SMP, you need to give her form SMP1, which allows her to apply for Maternity Allowance (MA).
- You need to find out about how to claim back the SMP you will need to pay (you claim back at least 92%).
- If SMP causes you cash flow problems, you can claim it back in advance.

There is an HM Revenue & Customs calculator and standard letters, as well as an SMP1 form, on the HMRC website:
- www.hmrc.gov.uk/employers
- HMRC Employer's Helpline 08457 143 143

Before your employee returns to work

- If she changes her mind about the date of return to work, she needs to give you 8 weeks notice of the change.
- If she will be breastfeeding on her return, you need to talk to her about her plans, such as expressing at work, and carry out a risk assessment.

[At the beginning] it was just knackering ... I used to go to work, come home, eat in silence, and collapse in to bed... And we had to do out-of-hours then, it was part of the contract. Actually later in the pregnancy, it was fine. I didn't change my number of sessions. At the end of the day, it all boils down to who you're working with, and what sort of relationship you've got with the partners in the practice.

GP

References

Department of Trade and Industry (2007) *Pregnancy and Work: What you need to know as an employer. Babies due on or after 1 April 2007*. Department of Trade and Industry, London.

Chapter 5

Academic medicine

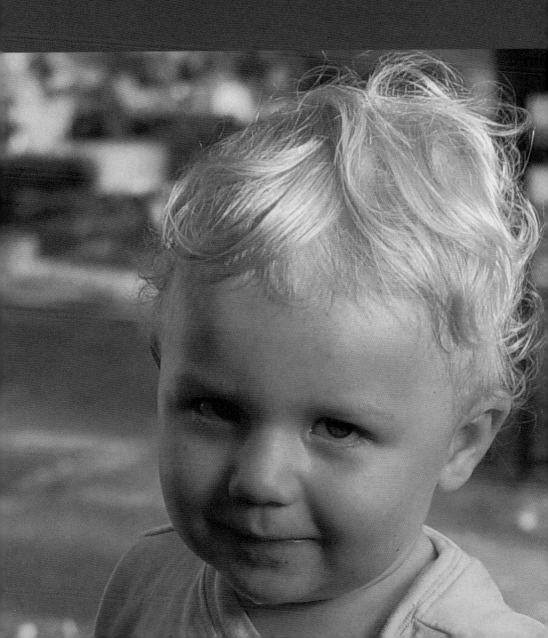

[My supervisor] said to me 'Now come on, academic medicine needs women, it needs you' but I just thought yes, but my children need me too.

ST haematology

Summary of academic training and positions under Modernising Medical Careers (MMC)

Academic training

Most of the positions are Fellowships; awards made for the purposes of the personal support of the doctor. Funding normally includes support for a research project or programme; the level of support increases with the level of seniority.

- *Academic Clinical Fellowship:* support, for up to 3 years, allowing the Fellow to undertake specialist clinical training, with about 25% of their time available for academic activities.

- *Training Fellowship:* normally for 3 years, allowing the fellow a period of usually full-time research, leading to publications and a doctorate (usually a PhD.)

- *Clinical Scientist Fellowship:* for a candidate who has a PhD or MD, and is close to finishing their specialist clinical training. Support is normally for up to 5 years, allowing the Fellow to continue their programme of research, while also working towards the CCT.

- *Senior Clinical Fellowship:* funding and research support for a doctor who already has extensive research experience, and is normally at award of, or after, a CCT. The doctor has limited clinical responsibility at consultant level, and often leads a small research team.

Academic positions

- *Clinical Lecturer:* a member of the university staff, who has a clinical contract (normally as an SpR) and who conducts research and teaches, while working towards the CCT.

- *Senior Lectureship, Readership or Professorship:* a more senior clinical academic position, usually a consultant who teaches and conducts research.

For more information, see the MMC website at http://www.mmc.nhs.uk

Research is the perfect time to get pregnant. You're more flexible, your learning is self directed, your pregnancy won't affect anyone around you, there's no locum to arrange, and if I needed a scan or an appointment, I just worked around it.

Consultant dermatologist

In one way, research was better [for hours] when we were doing the old hours … But then, I was doing 48 hours part-time as a registrar … So now, with the new hours, it may not be easier in terms of workload … Clinical research is hard work. We always used to say to women, 'Have your first baby when you're doing your research,' but I don't know whether you could advise that now.

Consultant surgeon

Maternity benefits

If you are employed by a university, on a university contract, it does not count as 'continuous service' under the NHS scheme (see Chapter 8) whether or not it was with an NHS honorary contract. If you have an NHS honorary contract, this period of employment doesn't count as a break in service.

My research was funded by the Wellcome Trust, and because I had been doing it for more than nine months when I went off on leave, they paid all my maternity leave … They paid me my full salary for sixteen weeks.

Consultant dermatologist

If you hold a University or an NHS honorary contract, you will not be covered by the NHS maternity scheme; you will be subject to the maternity leave scheme that is in operation at your place of employment. If there is not a maternity scheme, you will be subject to the statutory provisions (see Chapter 8).

If you have been in research and then return to hospital medicine, or general practice, be aware that you might not be entitled to maternity benefits for some time, as the university post will have broken the 'NHS continuous service.'

Working part time and doing research

My cells [that I was growing for my research project] didn't understand that I was working part time … Things would happen on days that I wasn't there, and nothing would happen on the days I was … It was really difficult.

ST haematology

You may or may not be able to do your research part time, depending on your funding, your boss, and the kind of research you're doing. You might prefer to return to academic work full time after you've had the baby, in order to complete the work in a shorter amount of time. As with all things related to pregnancy and leave, try and sort things out earlier rather than later, especially if you want to try and come back on a part-time basis.

> Our registrar has just returned after having a baby, she's come back part time. She had just started a research project, and it was very difficult for her, she had to go and see the professor and explain that she would be having a baby, so it all just fell by the way side really …

Consultant physician

References

British Medical Association (April 2007) *Maternity Leave (for NHS medical staff)*. Membership guidance note—NHS employment. British Medical Association, London.

UK Clinical Research Collaboration (March 2005) *Medically and Dentally Qualified Academic Staff: Recommendations for training the researchers and educators of the future*. Report of the Academic Careers Sub-Committee of MMC and the UK Clinical Research Collaboration.

Chapter 6

Pregnancy as an undergraduate

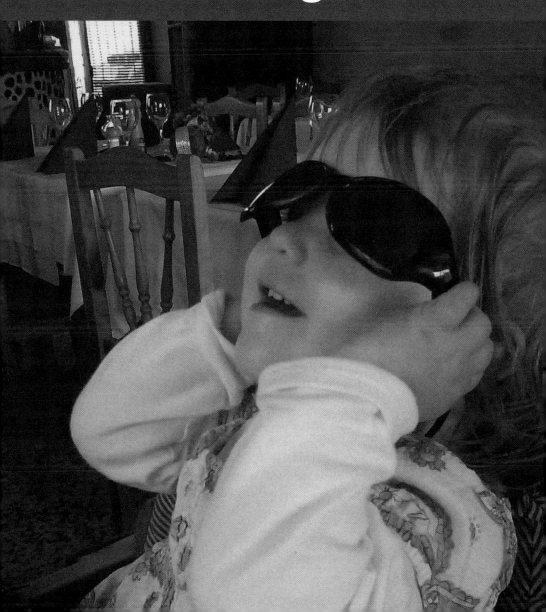

I used to really panic, in fact I got a bit depressed, because I thought I'd never, ever make it to being a doctor … Taking time off from university, to have my children, and taking things more slowly afterwards… But my Health Visitor was brilliant; she made me see the bigger picture. So now I'm a doctor, I'm doing fine, and my children are at school.

ST medicine

If you want to have children while you're still a student, it's worth contacting your college welfare services to find out if you'll be eligible for any financial help, and to find out the practicalities of taking a break in your studies. You might find it helpful to contact other women who have done the same thing, to find out what it was like and how they coped.

See Chapter 14 for information on childcare. One of your hospitals may have a staff nursery with graded fees based on how much you earn (or, in your case, don't earn). You may find that a childminder is a good value option, or an au pair could be right for you if you have the space.

I did my Finals, and then I had my baby a few weeks later at the beginning of July … The exams were good actually, it made me have something to look forward to, and I had a little person to talk to whilst I was revising!

FY1 doctor

We had some revision lectures just before our exams … I did notice that whenever I walked in the room there were whispers of 'Ooh look she's getting bigger' … But I felt like a bit of a celebrity!

FY1 doctor

Along with the Medical Women's Federation, the Medical Students Committee of the BMA recently carried out a survey, asking medical school deans what arrangements they have in place to help students who become pregnant during the undergraduate course. They state in their June 2005 report that provision varies across medical schools, and the MSC are working to develop guidelines that all medical schools should adhere to. In December 2006, they issued guidance for medical students with dependants. In summary, it states that:

- Female students do not qualify as 'employees' or 'workers,' therefore they cannot benefit from employment related rights.
- Even when you are on clinical placements, you might not necessarily qualify for those rights, as you are allocated the placements by the medical school and there is no direct legal or financial agreement between the hospital and the student.

- Therefore, the medical school has overall responsibility.
- Most medical schools have a case-by-case approach, rather than set guidelines.

Sources of support that may be useful to medical students who are planning a pregnancy, pregnant or with children may include:

- Medical school welfare officers/tutors
- University student union welfare and educational services
- University medical staff or medical centre
- The student's own GP
- Counselling services
- BMA Regional Services
- BMA Counselling Services.

To be honest, it [having children at school whilst I was a student] didn't really affect anything ... The most difficult attachment was surgery, because we had to be in at eight o'clock ... Sometimes I'd have to be late for surgery, and I'd have to clear that first ... They were actually fine about it.

Medical Student

Tell someone senior, even if you don't tell anyone else for a long time, as soon as you know that you're pregnant. Then you can at least get the ball rolling in terms of finding out how you're going to manage, what will happen to your course, exams etc., while you're deciding what to do. Remember that senior tutors at medical school have a great deal of experience with students; nothing shocks them, and you might not be the first student to tell them about a pregnancy. They will be delighted for you, and it is their job to help you complete your course.

Students should have a personal (sometimes called pastoral) tutor; they are usually one of the lecturers, and you should be able to go to them with problems relating to your study, or your personal life. If you don't get on with them, or if you don't feel comfortable talking to them (you may be terrified of them, or you may not want them to know that you're pregnant) you should be able to talk to one of the other senior tutors in confidence. Leave a message with their secretary, or contact them directly, explaining that you have an issue you don't want to discuss with your own tutor.

A lot of them [the other students] were really excited ... A lot of them were very curious ... There was a lot of curiosity about 'Why now?' ... But they can see I'm just so happy, so happy to have her, the main problem is me making other people really broody!

Medical student

> I took my maternity leave just before my Finals ... Then I came back and did my exams later on, when she was about one. When I came back after maternity leave I re-did some modules before I sat Finals, because I had forgotten everything ... I also had to do my elective [in a local hospital.]
>
> *FY1 doctor*

Full-time students may be able to claim social security benefits if they are responsible for children. You can claim income support if you are a lone parent, with a child under 16. Couples who are both full-time students and who are responsible for a child under the age of 19 may be able to claim income support during the summer holidays, as most student loans and grants don't cover the summer break; contact your local Department of Work and Pension (DWP) for more information.

If you are a full-time student with dependent children you should be able to claim Child Tax Credit, even though you're not working (see Chapter 19). If you are a student but your partner is working, you might be able to apply for Working Tax credit.

If you are a single parent, you may be able to claim Housing Benefit to help with your rent, and Council Tax Benefit if you are liable to pay council tax. These benefits are claimed from your Local Authority.

Disabled students may be able to claim Disability Living Allowance; contact the Benefits Enquiry Line on 0800 882 200.

You might also be eligible for help with NHS costs (dental treatment, prescriptions, sight tests, etc.). You can ask for a form from your local post office or GP surgery. Remember that if you are pregnant, and for the first year of your child's life, your prescriptions and dental treatment are free (see Chapter 19). Your child's prescriptions are also free.

> Of course, being a student, there was no such thing as maternity pay. My father was heavily involved ... I had to draw out loan payments;

Barclays' professional studies loans, grant payments and stuff … We didn't have a lot, and that was really hard.

FY1 doctor

> As soon as you know that you're taking time out to have a baby, write to the student loans company if you have a loan; they can then advise you about what happens to your loans if you take time out of your degree.

Other things to consider as a clinical student are the location of your hospital and GP placements. If you are starting medical school with children, or if you become pregnant during the course, let it be known earlier rather than later if you need placements to be near home; tutors will normally do their best to accommodate you, but as with all these things there needs to be a good line of communication in both directions, so speak up promptly if it looks like you're going to be struggling.

If you are pregnant or have children already, you should be able to arrange to do your elective at your local hospital; the medical school won't expect you to go to Papua New Guinea or Iraq, and just because you're close to home, it doesn't mean that you can't arrange a challenging and stimulating placement. If you can afford to take your family away with you, you should go for it and have a fantastic experience abroad!

The medical school arranged my clinical placements to be at X hospital, near my home, because I've got two children. Everyone [at the medical school] was really helpful.

ST medicine

Being a mum made me much less stressed about the whole starting work thing, because I had perspective.

FY1 doctor

References

http://www.bma.org.uk/ap.nsf/Content/mscdependentguidance
http://www.kcl.ac.uk/about/structure/admin/acareg/studentservices

Chapter 7

Know your rights: employment law

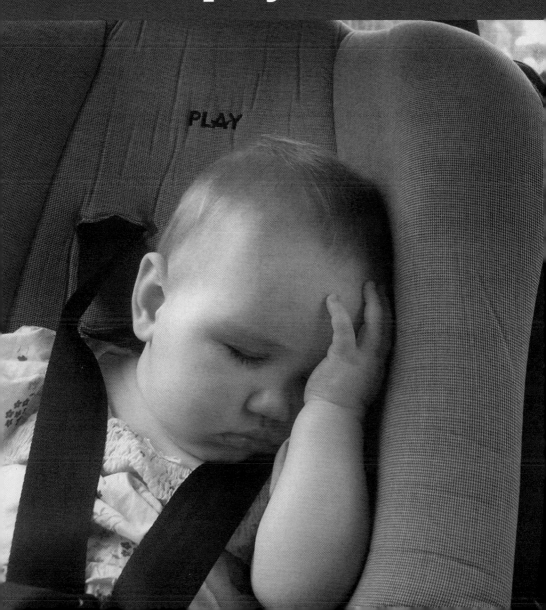

For the last three weeks, I had worked an illegal rota to cover someone who was away, plus a 20 hour weekend, and 50 hours this week. It was July, it was a heat-wave, and I was seven months pregnant … My longest break to eat, drink or pee was fifteen minutes, and I was on my feet all day, every day … It was Thursday, and I was due to work all weekend again on-call on the wards as a surgical house officer. I knew I couldn't take it, and I didn't want to phone in sick on Saturday morning and let the team down. So I went to see the consultant surgeon in charge of rotas to ask for help. I told him I was so sorry, but I just couldn't cope with doing the weekend. He said 'You've got me over a barrel. In any other country, you'd be given the sack.' I kept my composure as he signed the form, then I got up and left without saying a word. I refused to give him the satisfaction of seeing me cry.

ST medicine

There are two main Acts that give you rights during pregnancy and maternity leave. They are:

- Employment Rights Act 1996
- Sex Discrimination Act 1975.

The **Management of Health and Safety at Work Regulations 1999** require your employer to take certain steps to protect you when you are pregnant, breastfeeding, or have given birth in the last 6 months. **Note that they only apply if you have given your employer written notice of your pregnancy.**

Another girl has been through this hospital pregnant before, so I just have to do what she did.

ST surgery

The above regulations cover any female of childbearing age, who is pregnant, who could become pregnant, who has recently given birth, or who is breastfeeding. Of course, it would not be practical to try and adapt the working practices of doctors, just in case we were to become pregnant. You need to decide what would work best for you, at your specific time in your pregnancy, if you think you or your baby is being put at risk. Many doctors do things that are considered 'unsafe,' such as standing for long periods or not having a break. However, many doctors also feel that without the autonomy to dictate what is right for them, at this time in their training, they could not do their job properly. The key is to avoid truly risky behaviour, hopefully with the support of your team.

I had decided that I wasn't that keen on nailing long bones while I was pregnant, because of the radiation dose … I did one early on in the pregnancy, but the radiographer spent ages scanning around trying to find the tibia, and it scared me silly ... So I thought well, I'm not doing it again, but my boss did not agree ... He said the hospital wouldn't agree to monitor me for radiation dose... It only cost £35, so I said 'Look, I'll pay for the badge, I just want to know that I'm not getting zapped!' My boss said 'Look, you can't not nail ...' I said 'I can not nail, I'm trying to go down a line that's mutually acceptable, and I'm still doing my on calls and everything else ...' Then he went on holiday and left a patient who needed a nail for me to do ... He said 'Right, either you do it, or the patient will have to wait until I get back, and I know you wouldn't let the patient wait that long ...' I think he was waiting to see who cracked first ... I felt sorry for the patient, but I explained it all to him, and of course he was fine [about waiting] ... He said 'Oh well, you'd better get me a good book then!

Consultant orthopaedic surgeon

You are under no obligation to tell your employer that you are pregnant, or that you are breastfeeding. (You need to tell them in order to get maternity leave and pay though.) It is, of course, in your best interests to do so if you think you or the baby might be at risk. The best way to inform them is in writing, as until they have received written notification from you, they are not obliged to take any action to help you. It's prudent to enclose a copy of your Mat B1 certificate with this letter, and send a copy to HR (if you are in hospital).

Your employer has to carry out a risk assessment of your job, and this is supposed to be carried out in consultation with you. In practice, this doesn't always happen; in hospital, you may not be on very close terms with the consultant, or you may be the consultant; in which case, if you are the most senior consultant, you'll have to carry out the risk assessment with .... Yourself. Everybody knows that as doctors, we hate excessive paperwork. For many doctors, if they have a risk assessment at all, it consists of a quick chat with your partners/your consultant/other consultant colleagues, explaining that you won't be able to do specific tasks, such as working with the image intensifier in theatre, or staying in resus when portable X-rays are being done.

I'm working full time [at 25 weeks pregnant] which works out to be about 45 hours a week ... I'm still doing night shifts, starting at 5pm and finishing at 8am, but work has said that they'll stop me doing these in the last month I'm there ... I'm going to finish work 2 weeks before my due date. One thing that is specific for anaesthetics is the worry everyone has related to being pregnant, and working in orthopaedic theatres with X-rays. I asked the radiologist who did my scan, and he basically said the risk is miniscule, if you are wearing lead and not right underneath the X-ray machine. But I've noticed that despite my confidence in staying in the room while the X-ray is happening, a lot of theatre staff get quite twitchy, so unless there is a reason to be at the anaesthetic machine or doing something for the patient, I tend to leave the room now and stand in the anaesthetic room, still with my lead on. The other worry with anaesthetics is the use of nitrous oxide and anaesthetic gases … Nitrous oxide is going a bit out of fashion now anyway so I still use it, but only in specific circumstances and in quick procedures … It is supposedly associated with increased risk of miscarriages in the first trimester but the evidence isn't that conclusive.

ST anaesthetics

Risks identified by the HSE (see if you run out of fingers counting which ones apply to you):

- Lifting/carrying of heavy loads
- Standing or sitting for long lengths of time
- Exposure to infectious disease
- Exposure to lead
- Work-related stress
- Workstations and posture
- Exposure to radioactive material
- Other people's smoke in the workplace
- Threat of violence in the workplace
- Long working hours
- Excessively noisy workplaces.

According to the list above, 99% of doctors are 'at risk.' As discussed previously, the trick is to find a way of working that suits you, with the least amount of risk. You still have a job to do, and most of us love our jobs, and would hate to be demoted to more sedate, but boring, work.

Every time I tried to find out what my rights were, I was told 'We don't know,' by everybody … Why doesn't anybody know? If you work in other jobs, everyone knows what you can or can't do … As doctors, we are all too scared to say if we can't manage, we don't know what the right thing to do is.

ST paediatrics

The following actions are supposed to be monitored and reviewed in a regular basis, once you have notified your employer, in writing, that you are pregnant, have given birth in the last 6 months, or that you are breastfeeding:

1. Carry out a risk assessment that is specific to you, to take into account any medical advice from your GP or midwife.
2. If a risk is identified, can the risk be removed?

3. If the risk cannot be removed, can your working hours/working conditions be adjusted (at the same rate of pay)?
4. If not, can you be given suitable alternative work on the same terms and conditions (i.e. at the same rate of pay)?
5. If you cannot be given suitable alternative work, you must be suspended from work, on fully paid leave, for as long as is necessary to protect your health and safety, or that of your child.

Your employer must take into account any medical problems you have, such as a history of miscarriage, hypertension, etc. The risk assessment should be regularly reviewed, as the risks may differ at different times of the pregnancy. It is worth noting that you are officially entitled to more frequent rest breaks, but you may not get any official breaks during the day, and need to make sure you discuss this in the assessment.

> Being signed off sick from work may not resolve health problems, and may affect your maternity benefits. If you think that your work is making you ill, your employer should address the issue and take action as outlined above.

I didn't understand the NHS maternity regulations, as I had just arrived from abroad. I thought that I could ask my team if I could do some physically easier work, without having to carry the labour ward bleep. But I was just re-buffed; they said to me 'We don't know anything about these rules, because generally SHOs in this rotation don't tend to get pregnant.' But then I had pregnancy induced hypertension... I got a letter from my GP to say that I couldn't do nights and on calls, but the team was not very happy, and they asked me to go on leave. So I had three weeks off, then when [I went back and asked for help] they told me I would have to have a pay cut. So I just carried on, then I got ill again [with hypertension.]

ST paediatrics

Unless there is a specific risk identified, you must still work nights. If your GP or midwife supplies a medical certificate stating that you must not work nights, then your employer must offer you suitable alternative day work on the same terms and conditions, or if this is not possible, they must suspend you on full pay.

> It is the Trust's responsibility to arrange locum cover if you are not able to do your on-call duties.

Following childbirth, you are obliged to take 2 weeks off work. This is compulsory maternity leave. See Chapter 8 for more information on maternity leave.

You are entitled to paid time off to attend antenatal appointments; there is no limit as to the amount of time you can take off, on the advice of your GP or midwife.

HSE advice on breastfeeding (and see Chapter 13)

You are supposed to inform your employer in writing that you are breastfeeding. The HSE identifies the risks associated with breastfeeding as exposure to mercury, lead, or radioactive material; as a doctor, the most likely risk is not drinking enough during the day, and not having the time or place to express breast milk. Your employer is supposed to provide somewhere for breastfeeding mothers to rest. The HSE recommends that they also provide a private, safe environment for nursing mothers to express and store milk, but this is not a legal requirement. The HSE does not recommend that toilets are used for expressing milk.

If there is a problem: advice from the Department of Trade and Industry

- Try and talk to your employer first, to resolve the problem
- Talk to Occupational Health
- Contact the Health and Safety Executive www.hse.gov.uk
- You can get free confidential advice from the Acas helpline 08457 47 47 47 (in Northern Ireland the Labour Relations Agency on 028 9032 1442)
- There may be other sources of help, such as Citizen's Advice Bureau

Remember that you are protected from unfair treatment during your pregnancy or maternity leave.

The following is advice from the Equal Opportunities Commission, an independent, non-departmental public body, funded primarily by the government. You can visit their website at http://www.eoc.org.uk, or http://www.eoc-law.org.uk for specialist legal information. See the appendix at the back of the book for further contact details.

Pay during pregnancy and maternity leave

- You are entitled to paid time off for antenatal classes and appointments.
- You should still receive your pay rise every year during OML.

- Pension contributions should continue during OML.
- You will receive SMP (paid by your employer) or MA (paid by Social Security)—see Chapter 8 for more information.

Why can't people be more upfront about it? I mean, not only should you ring the BMA and check what you're entitled to before you get pregnant, but you should be able to ask your employer too ... Obviously everyone's worrying about jobs and the competitive nature of things ... But once you've got a job, why shouldn't we be able to ask other colleagues for advice? We spend all our lives working for the NHS, so we should be entitled to something.

GP

Your job during pregnancy and maternity leave

- In law, you cannot be dismissed because you are pregnant, or for reasons connected with your pregnancy or maternity leave.
- You have the right to be offered the same training and promotional opportunities as other staff while you are pregnant.
- You should be allowed to keep the same duties and responsibilities while you are pregnant.
- You should be allowed to return to the job that you left unless this is genuinely not possible, in which case you must be offered a suitable alternative.

Remember that in order to be protected by the law, and to receive the full extent of your rights, you have to tell your employer (in writing) that you are pregnant or breastfeeding.

If you think you have been treated unfairly at work because of your pregnancy, contact the EOC Helpline for information about what to do next:

- England: 0845 601 5901
- Wales: 029 2034 3552
- Scotland: 0141 245 1800.

The Sex Discrimination Act 1975

The Sex Discrimination Act 1975 makes it unlawful for employers to treat women or men less favourably because of their sex, in the area of employment. It applies to employees and to those applying for jobs.

Pregnancy and maternity discrimination can be in the following forms:

- Direct discrimination on the grounds of pregnancy (your employer treats you less favourably than they would have done, had you not become pregnant).
- Direct marriage discrimination (your employer passes you over for a job because you are married, and therefore more likely to want maternity leave in the future).

- Indirect sex discrimination (your employer applies a provision, such as never taking more than 3 months leave in order to achieve a good appraisal, which is more attainable by a man than a woman who might need maternity leave).
- Victimization, which comes about after you have asserted your rights as stated in the Sex Discrimination Act and are then treated less favourably, such as being demoted in your daily duties.

There is also indirect marriage discrimination, which is so complicated that I can't even begin to describe it. In a nutshell, you are protected by the SDA regardless of length of service, and regardless of the hours you work. It covers doctors who are self-employed as well as those who are employees, and in terms of general practice, the SDA covers discrimination by partners.

In order to claim sex discrimination, you must be able to show that:

1. But for your pregnancy, you would not have been treated badly.
2. The fact that you were pregnant was an effective cause of the way you were treated, even if it was not the sole reason for it.
3. The treatment that you received was detrimental to you.

The Employment Rights Act 1996

The above act protects pregnant employees and new and nursing mothers in regard to:

- Health and Safety.
- Unlawful dismissal because you are pregnant, or related to your maternity leave.
- Redundancy during your maternity leave.
- Changes to your job on your return from maternity leave.

As long as you have notified your employer correctly, in writing, you will be entitled to time off for antenatal care (including parenting classes and relaxation classes), 26 weeks of Ordinary Maternity Leave with all your normal terms and conditions except pay, plus 26 weeks of additional maternity leave. See Chapter 8 for a more detailed discussion of maternity leave, sickness during pregnancy and sick pay during pregnancy.

If you have suffered because your employer did not take appropriate action to protect you against risks, you can take a case under the Employment Rights Act. A failure to carry out a risk assessment, if you subsequently suffer, is automatically sex discrimination under the sex discrimination act. If your employer refuses to conduct a risk assessment at your request, and you think you will suffer as a result, contact the Health and Safety Executive for advice.

HSE Information Line 0845 345 0055

References

Department of Trade and Industry (2007) *Pregnancy and Work: What you need to know as an employer. Babies due on or after 1 April 2007*. Department of Trade and Industry, London.

Equal Opportunities Commission (2006) *Pregnancy and Maternity: Your rights*. Equal Opportunities Commission, Manchester.

Health and Safety Executive (2005) *A Guide for New and Expectant Mothers Who Work*. ISBN 0 7176 2614 8. Reprinted 07/05, Health and Safety Executive.

Chapter 8

Maternity leave
Part 1

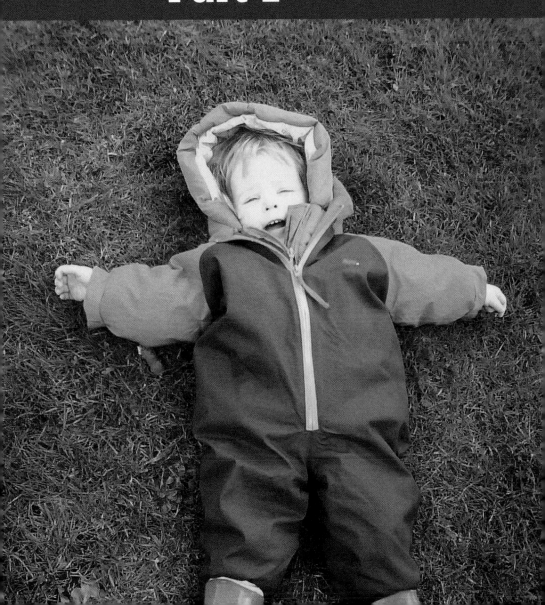

Part 1

Maternity leave for doctors: the NHS scheme

Like most things in the NHS, maternity leave is a complicated beast. The most important thing you can do, if you are planning a pregnancy or are pregnant already, is to get some individual advice, either through Human Resources (HR) or via the British Medical Association (BMA) if you're a member. If you are in general practice, your maternity rights should be laid out clearly in your contract, and they will vary depending on your position, local policy and practice. This chapter is a very rough guide, intended to give you an idea of what you might be entitled to, and to point you in the right direction for further help.

We should all sign contracts, whether we are planning a family or not, and whether we work in a hospital, general practice or a university. Your contract should mention something about maternity leave; if not, you need to clarify the situation before signing it (this sounds obvious, but is easy to miss in the hectic whirl of starting a new job).

Doctors working in hospitals, community health, and public health on standard contracts of employment should (but may not) be entitled to the NHS scheme. GPs employed by practices, or by primary care organizations, and sometimes salaried GPs should be covered by the scheme, if your contract of employment incorporated the National Terms and Conditions of Service.

> Some NHS trusts employ a Maternity Adviser in the Human Resources department, who will be available to discuss all aspects of maternity leave and pay.

Your maternity rights fall into four categories:

1. Time off work, with pay, for antenatal care.
2. Maternity leave (26 weeks of Ordinary Maternity Leave, plus 26 weeks of Additional Maternity Leave). This makes 52 weeks in total of leave, but not 52 weeks of pay.
3. Maternity pay.
4. Protection against unfair treatment or dismissal.

The two maternity benefits available to you are:

1. Statutory Maternity Pay (SMP), paid by your employer, or
2. Maternity Allowance (MA), paid by the Department for Work and Pensions.

Who is eligible for maternity leave?

Maternity leave is covered by the Employment Rights Act 1996. It states that by the time you are about 25 weeks pregnant (by the end of the 15th week before the expected week of childbirth) you must notify your employer of your pregnancy, the expected week of childbirth, and when you intend your maternity leave to start. You can change this date, as long as you give your employer 28 days notice. You can take your maternity leave any time from the 11th week before the week in which the baby is due, when you are about 29 weeks pregnant. You are entitled to 26 weeks of Ordinary Maternity Leave plus 26 weeks of Additional Maternity Leave.

BMA members can access the maternity leave calculator via the BMA website (once you have logged in as a member, search for 'maternity calculator' and enter your Estimated Delivery Date). It assists the pregnant brain by telling you exactly which date you should have told your employer by, the earliest date you can start your maternity leave, etc.

- www.bma.org.uk

If you are a doctor, working under the NHS scheme either part-time or full-time, you will be entitled to paid and unpaid maternity leave if:

- You intend to return to work for the NHS, either full-time or part-time, for a minimum of 3 months full time or part time equivalent.
- You have worked for 12 continuous months, without a break of more than 3 months, with one or more NHS employers at the beginning of the 11th week before the expected week of childbirth (by the time you are about 28 weeks pregnant, you will have worked in the NHS for a year).
- You tell your employer in writing before the end of the 15th week before your expected date of childbirth (by the time you are about 24 weeks pregnant). There are situations in which you can tell your employer later, if it was not practical beforehand. If you are in a hospital post, you should write to your HR department and your consultant if you are a junior. 'Your employer' is the NHS, but if you are changing jobs before you have the baby, you are probably safest writing to HR and the consultant at your new job, as well as at your existing job, just to cover everything.

In your letter, you should write the following:

1. That you intend to take maternity leave.
2. The date you want your maternity leave to start (don't worry if you don't know yet; this date can be changed, ideally with 28 days notice, but less if this is not practical).
3. That you have every intention of returning to work for the NHS for at least 3 months after your maternity leave.
4. You also need to supply a Mat B1 form from your midwife or GP, stating your Estimated Date of Delivery (EDD).

....

This is a form that will be given to you by your midwife/GP/consultant, usually after your 12-week scan, which will state your Estimated Delivery Date (EDD).

Make sure you take a few photocopies, in case HR loses it, you are changing jobs part-way through your pregnancy, or the dog eats it.

'With one or more NHS employers?'

These include health authorities, NHS boards, NHS trusts, primary care trusts, and the Northern Ireland Health Service.

'Without a break of more than three months?'

If you were off work for less than 3 months, this doesn't affect 'continuous service', but it doesn't count as service. So you will need to have been working in the NHS for longer than 12 months in total.

There are other situations where it doesn't matter that you weren't employed by the NHS, but again these don't count as service:

1. If you were employed under the terms of an honorary contract.
2. If you did a locum as a GP that was less than 12 months.
3. Up to 12 months working abroad, but only if it was part of postgraduate training programme, and was done on the advice of a dean/college/faculty adviser in your speciality.
4. Up to 12 months doing voluntary service overseas with 'a recognized international relief organisation', such as VSO. This can apparently be extended to a further 12 months but is 'at the discretion of the employer,' so be careful.
5. Absence on an 'employment break scheme'.
6. Absence on maternity leave if it was provided for on the NHS scheme above, whether it was paid or unpaid.

Be aware though that the goalposts can move. Apparently employers can, at their own discretion, extend the 12-month period. How much more confusing can it get?

What is my Expected Week of Childbirth (EWC)?

This is defined as the week, beginning with midnight between Saturday and Sunday, in which it is expected that you will give birth.

If your contract is due to end after the 11th week before the EWC (i.e. after you are about 28 weeks pregnant):

- As long as you are eligible as outlined above, your contract will be extended so that you can receive your 26 weeks paid maternity leave (see later).
- If you want to take your 26 weeks unpaid maternity leave it does not count as a break in service, and you will not have to repay your maternity leave because you can't return to your post.

How much maternity pay will I get?

The general rule is, from April 2007:

- 26 weeks of paid maternity leave plus 26 weeks of unpaid maternity leave.
- You will get 8 weeks of full pay, less SMP or MA (see below).
- You will then get 18 weeks of half pay, plus any SMP or MA, as long as the total amount does not exceed your normal full pay.

How is my 'pay' calculated?

Your maternity pay is calculated on your average weekly earnings for the 8 weeks ending with the qualifying week. The qualifying week is the 15th week before the EWC, i.e. your pay between about 16 and 24 weeks of your pregnancy.

It is normally based on your gross earnings, including London weightings and banding supplements.

If you are concerned that your pay will drop dramatically half way through your leave, it should be possible to arrange for you to be paid a fixed amount per month. Talk to your employer to see if you can receive a set sum over 6 months instead.

What if I changed Trusts during my pregnancy?

- If you qualify for the NHS scheme, but do not have 26 weeks continuous service with the same Trust by the time you reach the qualifying week (the 15th week before the EWC, i.e. when you are about 24 weeks pregnant) you still get maternity pay. **You will still get the full amount, but part of it needs to be claimed by you from the state (the Benefits Agency),** rather than your employer claiming it for you.

- Your employer will not be able to claim back SMP (see below) from the state.
- This means that you need to claim Maternity Allowance (see below) directly from the Benefits Agency.

If you have never had a reason to deal with the Benefits Agency before, prepare yourself for an organization that can seem even more disorganized than the NHS. As stated above, you only need to claim from the Benefits Agency if you change Trusts.

Statutory Maternity Pay

Unless you have changed Trusts during your pregnancy (see above), the SMP forms part of your maternity pay. Like the rest of your maternity pay, it is paid to you directly by your employer, but your employer then claims it back from the Inland Revenue.

You get SMP for a maximum of 39 weeks. You can still get SMP if you don't plan to go back to work. You don't have to pay SMP back if you decide not to return to work.

- For the first 6 weeks, you get 90% of your average weekly pay.
- After that, you will get the basic rate of SMP, which is £112.75 per week for 33 weeks.
- If 90% of your average pay is less than £112.75, then you will receive that amount instead.
- Your employer will deduct tax and National Insurance in the usual way; your SMP is normally paid in the same way as your salary, and you should receive a printed pay slip as normal.

Your SMP can be paid to you from 11 weeks before the expected week of childbirth, i.e. when you are about 29 weeks pregnant. You need to inform your employer in writing at least 28 days before you want the SMP to start of the date you want to start your pay. Send your MatB1 certificate with the letter (after you've taken a few photocopies). Once you inform your employer about when you want your pay to start, you are not allowed to change your mind.

Go to the Department for Work and Pensions site for detailed information on maternity benefits:
- http://www.dwp.gov.uk/advisers/ni17a

Maternity Allowance

You may be entitled to this if you can't get SMP, for example if you have changed Trusts during your pregnancy. You can also claim MA if you are self-employed. You must have worked in at least 26 of the 66 weeks before your expected week of childbirth. You must have earned at least £30 per week for 13 weeks. You may therefore be able to claim MA if you are a student, providing you have been doing part-time work that wasn't just a bar job with cash in hand. Choose the weeks in which you earned the most money; you may have gone up grades, changed specialities, or changed banding.

MA is paid at £112.75 a week, or 90% of your average earnings if this is less, for 26 weeks. MA is not liable to income tax or NI contributions.

- MA is only paid for weeks when you are not at work.
- The earliest you can claim it is 15 weeks before your baby is due, when you are about 25 weeks pregnant.
- The earliest it can start is 11 weeks before your baby is due, when you are about 29 weeks pregnant.
- The latest it can start is your EWC.

It is probably good practice for doctors to have an insight into the world of the Benefits office, if you haven't already. Never again will you criticize your hospital switchboard, however bad it is, and never again will you moan about filling in forms at work—the MA form goes on for ever, and I congratulate you if you can fill it all in without ripping it to shreds and hurling it out of the window. To get hold of the form, you need to contact your local Jobcentre Plus. If you are unsure whether you can claim MA or not, it is worth filling out the form anyway, with gritted teeth, as the friendly staff will calculate whether you are entitled or not.

- **If you don't claim within 3 months of giving birth, you may lose the benefit.** Remember that once the baby arrives, you will have no patience/time/will to fill the form out, so you should ideally do it before giving birth.
- The form you require is **MA1**.
- You can get MA1 from any Jobcentre Plus, but they may have copies at your antenatal clinic.
- You send the completed form to the Jobcentre Plus, along with your MAT B1 (making sure you have photocopied it).
- You must also send form **SMP1** from your employer. This is a form that shows why you don't qualify for SMP. Give your employer some notice, as it may take a while to organize the form, and as always photocopy it before sending it.
- **MA1 needs to be sent in as soon as you are 26 weeks pregnant.** The other paperwork can be sent on at a later date, but it's probably easier to send it all together.
- It is probably easiest to get MA paid directly into your bank account, rather than faffing around with a book of orders that you need to cash.

Incapacity Benefit (IB)

Don't panic; this does not mean you are incapable. IB is for women who can't get SMP or MA. If your MA form gets processed and it turns out that you can't get MA, they will automatically assess you for IB. Like being a house officer though, don't forget to chase up those results, as sometimes they forget.

To be eligible for IB you must have paid enough National Insurance contributions in earlier tax years.

- It is about £60–70 per week.
- It is paid from 6 weeks before your baby is due, until 2 weeks after your baby is born.

Sickness before maternity leave starts

If you have to go off sick, with a pregnancy-related illness it can affect your maternity leave:

- If it is during the last 4 weeks before the EWC, your maternity leave will start at the beginning of the fourth week before the EWC, or the beginning of the next week after you the week you last worked in, whichever is later. In plain English, you will be starting your maternity leave if you go off sick (with a pregnancy related illness) in the last 4 weeks of your pregnancy.
- If you are off sick before the last 4 weeks before the EWC, it is treated as normal sick leave, and paid as such.
- If there is the occasional day of sickness in the last month, it can be disregarded by the employer if they wish, and you can start your maternity leave on the date you previously wanted to.
- If your sickness is not related to pregnancy, your normal sick leave provisions apply until the date which you notified for the start of your maternity leave.

Premature babies

If your baby is born alive prematurely, you are entitled to the same amount of maternity leave and pay as if the baby was born at full term.

If the baby is born before the 11th week before the EWC, and you were at work during the actual week of childbirth, your maternity leave will start on the first day of your absence from work.

If you were off work sick (classed as certified sickness, i.e. with a sick note) during the week you gave birth, your maternity leave will start at the beginning of your week of childbirth.

If your baby is born alive before the 11th week before the EWC, you are entitled to split your maternity leave—you can take 2 weeks (or more) immediately after the birth, then the rest of your leave following the baby's discharge from hospital.

Miscarriage

If you have a miscarriage before the 25th week of pregnancy, normal sick leave provisions will apply.

Maternity leave and pay for doctors working in general practice

> Women need to look at the Partnership agreement, so carefully, and just see what it says ... The maternity rights will reflect on everything else that practice stands for, so make sure you read them carefully.
>
> *GP*

ST3 General Practice (GP Registrars)

During the hospital part of your VTS scheme, you are employed by the NHS and as such are entitled to the maternity benefits outlined above. Once you become an ST3, you are on a contract of employment with the training practice rather than the NHS, but it is generally agreed that you are still entitled to the NHS scheme. Check your contract, and discuss it with your trainer if you're not sure of your entitlements.

In terms of length of service, your time spent as an ST3 in general practice counts for length of service requirements.

As an ST3 (GP), you should be entitled to 8 weeks full pay, less SMP or MA, plus 14 weeks half pay plus any SMP or MA (as long as the total doesn't exceed full pay,) then 4 weeks at the standard rate of SMP or MA.

> Initially the plan was to get my training out of the way ... But I didn't want to go into a partnership straight away. And I realized that I might have to work a full 12 months first in order to get any maternity pay, which would delay it even more ... And because my training would have finished, there wouldn't be the opportunity of flexi-training ... It would be at the discretion of the practice, whether to allow me to come back part time or not. You're protected whilst you're training, you've got more options.
>
> *ST3 General Practice*

Salaried GPs

Salaried GPs may be entitled to both paid and unpaid maternity leave, but the details should be outlined in the individual's contract, and like all things maternity, never assume anything. The BMA has some good links on its website (www.bma.org.uk) and you can search for 'salaried GPs.' If it seems like I'm confused myself with this one, then I am; it looks complicated.

GP partners

GP partners will have their maternity leave and pay outlined in their individual contract. The amount of maternity pay awarded can vary wildly, from no pay at all, to full pay for 6 months.

> Once you become a Partner, you enter into a partnership agreement, which is drawn up between the partners, and can of course say anything it wants … So it may say that you are entitled to no maternity pay … In theory they should be offering what the NHS might offer as standard … A lot of Partnerships offer a much better arrangement [than in the NHS.]
>
> *GP*

> If the PCT don't cough up the money [for our partner who is currently pregnant] … Well, it's going to be hard … Of course, she'll get her full pay, because that's what's in the partnership agreement, but if the PCT won't pay, then that's a significant amount of money that we have to find from somewhere … And some practices may not have planned for this event … At the end of the day, either you don't get a locum in and the other partners take up the slack, or you get a locum in and everyone takes a drop in pay.
>
> *GP*

> When I was pregnant, we were still under the old contract … The new contract came in while I was on maternity leave… The new GP contract doesn't stipulate anywhere about what rights GPs should have in terms of GP partners. The Red Book (the old contract) stated that the Health Authority had to pay the practice maternity leave pay… Based on whether you were full-time/half-time …. It equated to about £960 a week. But now, what's happened is that there are no guidelines. PCTs now, they have a budget, which they can use, at their discretion if they wish, for things like covering maternity leave, sick leave.
>
> *GP*

Doctors who adopt a child

The Paternity and Adoption Leave Regulations (2002) cover families who adopted children after 6 April 2003. If you adopt a child, you can take 26 weeks of Ordinary Adoption Leave (OAL) and 26 weeks of Additional Adoption Leave (AAL).

If you are part of a couple, then only one of you can claim ordinary adoption leave. The other half of the couple may be entitled to paternity leave and pay.

In order to qualify for OAL, you must be the child's adopter, have been continuously employed for at least 26 weeks (ending with the week in which you were matched with the child), and notified the agency that you agree that the child should be placed with you on the date of placement.

If you adopt more than one child, as part of the same arrangement, you are only entitled to one period of OAL. The OAL begins on a date chosen by you.

References

British Medical Association (April 2007) *Maternity Leave (for NHS staff)*. Membership Guidance Note—NHS employment. British Medical Association, London.

Department of Health (2007) *Birth to Five*. Department of Health Publications, London.

Health and Safety Executive (2003) *A Guide for New and Expectant Mothers Who Work*, INDG373. Reprinted 07/05. HSE Books, London.

http://www.bma.org.uk/ap.nsf/Content/FocusSalariedGps0604#Maternityleavebenefits (advice for salaried GPs)

http://www.direct.gov.uk

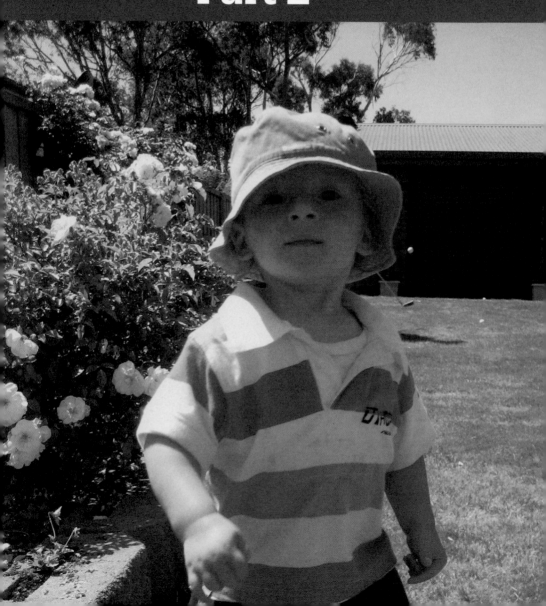

Maternity leave
Part 2

Part 2

Everyone says to me it'll be difficult to tell how much time I'm going to need off before I've had the baby, it's best to wait and see, and then make decisions.

GP

To return or not to return: the logistics

You don't need to give your employer notice if you intend to return to work immediately after your period of Additional Maternity Leave; see Chapter 8 Part One for more details on Ordinary and Additional Maternity Leave. If you want to return to work before the end of your Ordinary, or Additional, Maternity Leave entitlement, you need to give your employer 8 weeks notice. The thought of going back to work might fill you with horror, or fill you with excitement, but either way remember that 8 weeks is a long time in a baby's life. If you're nervous, and it seems too soon to be contacting work and making arrangements, bear in mind that in 8 weeks from now your baby will be a different person; more independent and more able to take on the fun challenges of days with a nanny or at nursery.

> If you are unable to return to work when you had planned, due to sickness, normal sick leave and pay arrangements apply. You need to get a sick note from your doctor and send it to work.

When you return after maternity leave, you are entitled to return to the same job you were in before. The exception is if you return after your full 12 months, where it might not be practical to fit you back into the same job; but you should be offered a job that is on the same terms and conditions as your previous one.

I was due to get my CCST the same week as she was due, there was no planning there; as my CCST came up, and I took maternity leave, I wasn't granted the six month extension period of grace that one would normally have had ... My maternity leave counted as my period of grace, which I felt aggrieved about ... I did write a letter [to complain], but I never posted it, because I didn't want to sound like a bitter woman! I was lucky though; the colleagues I was working with at that time were keen to have me back as a part time consultant; they'd managed to scrabble some money together, so I had about seven months of maternity leave, and at that point the post came up, and it worked out ok.

Consultant physician

> If you decide not to go back to work after maternity leave, you need to give notice of termination as outlined in your contract of employment.

If you know before you go on maternity leave that you don't want to go back to work, you can still claim SMP and you don't have to pay it back afterwards. If, after having your baby, you decide not to return to work, tell your employer in writing. If they thought you were returning to work, and you don't go back within 15 months of starting your maternity leave, you may have to repay all your maternity pay (less any SMP or MA you might have been paid). Your employer does have the ability to waive this, if they think that paying the money back would cause you 'undue hardship or distress.'

Making the decision not to return to work won't be easy. You worked hard for your career before you had children, and although the thought of returning might be daunting, it's amazing how quickly you can slot back into the role of being a doctor. If you were genuinely unhappy as a doctor before you had a baby, then you're probably making the right decision now. But if you enjoyed your job, and it's the thought of being away from your baby that's stopping you returning, it might be worth asking if you can spend some time 'observing' at work, as an unpaid presence on the ward or in the surgery, like a clinical attachment. Just being back at work, with your colleagues, and having some child-free time to yourself to do what you were trained to do, might make the transition easier.

> It was awful [being on maternity leave] ... I lost my identity completely. I work under my maiden name, but I had moved, and up here, nobody knew me as X, they all knew me as Mrs Y ... And that was a name I'd never used ... And I was either A's wife, or the baby's mother ... I didn't know anybody here at all ... Going back to work was just lovely, because at last I was back doing something that I knew how to do ... I thought great, I'm actually trained to do this.
>
> *Consultant surgeon*

There are organizations run by trained doctors, such as Doctors for Doctors, who may be able to help if you're feeling torn. See Appendix 1 in this book (section on 'Health—You.')

Jobseeker's Allowance

If you really hated being a doctor, and you need to find some other form of work, then you may be able to claim Jobseeker's Allowance (JSA). You would have to show that you had 'just cause' for voluntarily leaving your job as a doctor though, and you must be available for work for at least 16 hours a week. You may be able to claim for up to 6 months, but it's not a huge amount, about £50 a week. If you want to make an enquiry, then you need to visit your local Jobcentre Plus.

Planning your return

If you get the chance, and you don't have live-in childcare, you might want to do a 'dummy run' to work before your first day. Get everything ready the night before and plan how you're going to get to nursery or the childminder's. Get up at the same time you'll need to once you've started work, and get ready with the baby. Some people find it easier to set the alarm really early and get showered and dressed before the baby wakes up, others find it easier to be woken up by the baby and get ready together. Toddlers are usually quite happy to race around, yanking the shower curtain down and putting toys down the toilet while you try and get ready, but a smaller baby might need more attention. Check that your work clothes still fit you, and don't get depressed if they don't, then have breakfast and head off 'to work.' It might seem like a very stressful thing to do, but it might help you iron out some problems before you actually have to do it. If the traffic was awful, and the baby hated being in the car, is public transport another option? If the buses were all too full to get on with a buggy, can you go by car? Was there anywhere to park at the nursery? If you return home at 10 a.m. frazzled and with a migraine, remember that it won't always seem this stressful, and you'll get used to it more quickly than you can imagine.

Remember that most childcare providers need a period of 'settling in' (see Chapter 14 for more details). This can take several weeks, especially with a nursery, so make sure you don't leave it until the last minute. The very first time I left my baby with the childminder, my husband and I set off to the shops for some reckless shopping and eating, only to find that we sat and ate sushi in silence, then raced back to the baby as soon as my husband gave in to my pleas. We arrived to find her playing happily, and she was most annoyed to be taken home again. I think the moral of this story is; enjoy your sushi. The baby will be having a brilliant time.

References

British Medical Association (April 2007) *Maternity Leave (for NHS staff)*. Membership Guidance Note—NHS employment. British Medical Association, London.

Department of Health (2007) *Birth to Five*. Department of Health Publications, London.

Chapter 9

Before the baby arrives

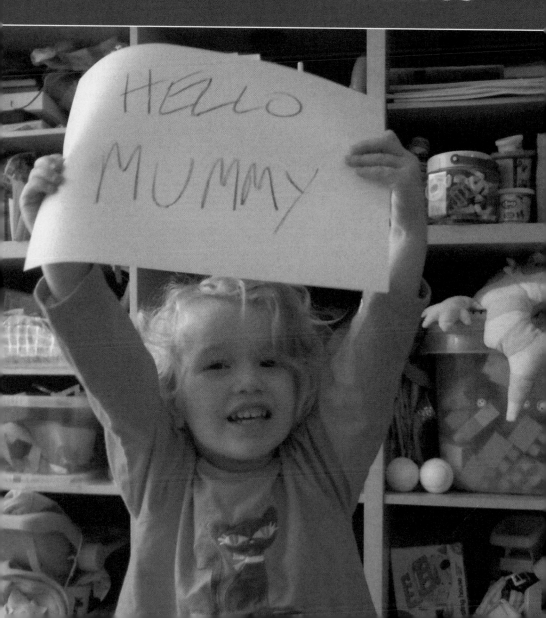

I didn't really know what to do with myself ... I was nesting I suppose, doing lots of sorting, but I didn't know many people outside work.

I started going to an aquanatal group, and I met another doctor, a GP. We had the same midwife, and after the baby was born, I asked to be put in touch with her; she gave me her phone number ... We actually met a lot of women who were doctors, and we developed quite a good social group!

Consultant physician

Congratulations, you have finished work! Your days of investigating patients are soon to be replaced by days of working out how the car seat fits in your car (or doesn't). Now is the time to get some rest, some sleep, and eat lots of cakes.

Suddenly you have all the time in the world, but you may notice that your medical friends, whom you would love to spend time with, are unavailable. They are still at work, doing evening surgery or sitting in the Grand Round every time you call. The solution, however much it may fill you with horror, is to make friends with some local women who are also pregnant. I say horror, because you probably have lots of great friends already, and you may feel this is entirely unnecessary, but it really does make a difference. Being pregnant, giving birth, and living with a baby are unique life experiences, and you will need people who know what you're going through, and who are around to meet up for coffee when it's all too much at 10 a.m. when all your old friends are busy at work. Every woman has bad days, and much as your friends love you, unless they have a child they won't know what you're going through. You'll also find that on bad days, when you just can't bear the stress of getting ready to leave the house, your baby is suddenly an angel once in the company of other mums and babies, as if they too needed to get away from it all.

My mum suggested that I join a local National Childbirth Trust (NCT) group, but I am ashamed to say that, for whatever reason, I had visions of women with hairy armpits giving birth in their back gardens. I dreaded the first meeting, and considered leaving my husband, with his 'straight-to-the-point what the hell are you daft mad women talking about' comments, at home. I was delighted to be proven wrong, and from the first meeting I knew I had done the right thing. Our teacher was incredible, and there was no hint of anti-medicalization of childbirth. All the options were discussed, and I realized that as a doctor I knew only a very small amount. The friends I made at the classes are very dear to me, as they went through an amazing life experience at the same time, and I'm very glad I met them. If you do decide to join the NCT, bear in mind that classes are very popular, and you may have to book in your first trimester just to guarantee a place. If you can't afford to join an organized group, or don't want to, don't worry. You'll get plenty of opportunity to meet other mums at your baby clinic (see Chapter 11), or your health visitor can put you in touch with local people.

National Childbirth Trust (NCT)

The NCT is a charity that has branches in every part of the UK. Its aim is to help all parents have '... An experience of pregnancy, birth and early parenthood that enriches their lives and gives them confidence in being a parent.'

As well as holding great second-hand sales where you can pick up anything from nearly new clothes to cots (if you arrive early), they hold antenatal classes, which are not only an excellent introduction to parenthood, but will enable you to meet other mums (and dads)-to-be in your area.

To find out about dates and locations of second hand sales, go to the NCT website and click on NEWS: to book classes: 0870 444 8707

They also run new baby groups, open house get-togethers, support for dads, and groups for working parents.

Bras for pregnancy and breastfeeding: 0870 112 1120 for a free catalogue, or order online at http://www.nctsales.co.uk

To join the NCT costs £36, call 0870 990 8040.

All members get a newsletter with local information and events listings:

• http://www.nctpregnancyandbabycare.com

Having sex while you're pregnant

Having sex is safe during pregnancy, but if you have some bleeding in early pregnancy, you may be advised not to have sex for a while.

You may, after a busy day at work, feel too exhausted/fat/sick to contemplate having sex. This is completely normal, and most relationships adapt to a new balance. There is evidence that domestic violence increases during pregnancy, and if you are feeling at risk, there are people who can help you; I'm not suggesting that this is related to a lack of sexual intimacy, but even a normal pregnancy can put the best relationship under strain at times.

If your relationship comes under strain during your pregnancy, and you think you might benefit from counselling, contact Relate (http://www.relate.org.uk to find your nearest centre).

Freephone 24 hour National Domestic Violence Helpline 0808 2000 247

If you're taking a long period of time off for maternity leave, and you stop working well before the baby is due, you may be lucky enough to squeeze in a mini-break, to get some well earned rest.

After 28 weeks all airlines will need a letter from your GP or obstetrician that states that you are fit to travel, and confirms your Estimated Date of Delivery. Each airline has its own rules, so check before you fly, but scheduled airlines may let women fly up to about 34 weeks (remember that if you fly out at 34 weeks to Albania, you may be stuck in Albania for your delivery at 40 weeks). Make sure you inform your travel insurance company; some will not cover you during the last couple of months of pregnancy.

> My husband and I took two months off work, and flew out to Hong Kong when I was thirty two weeks pregnant … We spent two months travelling back to the UK overland, on the Trans Mongolian Railway, fifteen thousand miles!
>
> *Consultant dermatologist*

Most airlines allow pregnant women to fly up to and including the 36th week, provided the pregnancy has been straightforward. The regulatory body for travel agents, IATA, says that pregnant women can fly in weeks 36–38 as long as the flying time doesn't exceed 4 hours, but you obviously need to check this. Eurostar and Eurotunnel have no restrictions. Airlines normally refuse to fly pregnant women who have previously given birth prematurely.

- http://www.netdoctor.co.uk/travel/diseases/pregnancy_and_travel.htm
- http://www.cheapflights.co.uk/travel-tips/travelling-while-pregnant.html

For information on when different airlines will let you fly:

- http://airtravel.about.com/cs/safetysecurity/a/pregflyer2_2.htm

You also need to use these precious weeks (or days) before delivery to go shopping. You will not be allowed to drive your baby home from hospital unless you have an appropriate car seat; so unless you want your other half to do a mercy dash to Mothercare while you're waiting in the 'departure lounge', you need to get organized beforehand.

Since September 2006, children who are either less than 135 cm tall or aged under 12 years, must travel in an appropriate child restraint in a car. You can't buy a second hand car seat; the car may have been involved in an accident.

Rear-facing car seats can only be used in the front seat if any airbag present has been deactivated.

To add to your stress, not all car seats fit all cars; you may need to consult your car manufacturer. Britax have devised a web site that allows you to check which seats will fit your car (http://www.britax.co.uk) or go to http://www.mothercare.com for vehicle compatibility listings, but most shops will allow you to try the car seat out in your car before you buy it.

A guide to car seats for people who have a PhD

1. **Infant carrier car seats**: from birth to about 15 months. These are supposed to be lightweight so you can carry them around (apart from the fact they contain a big lump of a baby) and face backwards. Some prams have a removable infant carrier. Great for when the baby is asleep and you need to move them in and out of the car.

2. **Isofix infant carriers**: from birth to about 15 months. These seats can face forwards or backwards, but they clip on to a base that is anchored in your car; from February 2006, all new cars will have special anchorage points.

3. **Combination car seats**: from birth to 4 years. For the first 15 months or so, the baby faces backwards. It then becomes a forward facing system.

4. **Forward facing car seats**: from 9 months to 4 years.

5. **Highback booster seats with integral harnesses**: 9 months–4 years.

6. **Highback boosters without harnesses and booster seats**: from 4 to 11 years

Except for the Isofix seats, all car seats are held in place by your car seat belt.

- http://www.mothercare.com has more details
- http://www.which.co.uk for unbiased advice and information on car seats.

If you thought buying a car was complicated and expensive, just wait until you have to choose a pram. My first car, a Ford Escort with leopard print seats, cost £400 from a dodgy bloke in Slough. As a result, I refused to spend anything like that amount on my first pram, but if you have money to burn, you can really go to town.

Prams: the problem with too many choices

Tip: It is possible to find a pram that will last your baby from birth until they are fully mobile. Think about how often you use public transport, if at all, how many steps you have to lug the pram up, whether you need an integral car seat, and whether you can afford to upgrade your buggy as the baby grows.

The last minute dash to Mothercare before you go into labour can be tricky. The trouble is that, once the baby arrives, you may not have time to go shopping for baby blankets and nappies, so it's best to stock up. My mum steered me around the shop, piling in babygros and hats, while I stared, transfixed, at the small babies around me, and then started crying in the maternity bra section.

1. **2-in-1 or 3-in-1 pram**: from birth or 6 months. Look like the traditional pram, usually allow the baby to face you. The baby can usually lie flat. It may have a 'carry cot' that lifts off separately. Can include a car seat, but as a result are often pricey and heavy. Don't even think about getting on a crowded bus with one.

2. **Three-wheeler**: from birth or 6 months. Great for 'off-roading' or jogging around the park if you're mad. May also incorporate a car seat or carry cot, and may allow the baby to face you. Usually more expensive.

3. **Forward facing**: from birth. Usually allow the baby to lie flat, but the seat tends to face away from you. This can be daunting when your baby is tiny, but before long the baby will be much more interested in looking at the world ahead than at you.

4. **Stroller**: from birth, 3 or 6 months. These are usually light and easy to transport/fold. Great if you use public transport a lot, or for going on holiday.

5. **Tandems/twin seaters**: some are for twins; some are for two children of different ages. Again, don't attempt the rush hour on public transport.

So there's me, going round Mothercare, and it suddenly hit me, I haven't got a clue … I know absolutely nothing about all this stuff …

ST A&E

I blamed it on the hormones, but it was a necessary evil; at the very least you need to have a bag ready for when you go into hospital. Some women manage to organize this at about 20 weeks gestation, but a few days before I was due I was still scratching my head and wondering what on earth I needed. Here are some of the essentials for 'The hospital bag'.

The hospital bag

- Nappies
- Cotton wool
- Vaseline
- Aqueous cream/other moisturizer
- *For baby*: short-sleeved vests, babygros/ sleepsuits, blanket, hats, mittens, towels, changing mat
- *For you*: nightie or pyjamas, breast pads, lip balm, spare underwear, sanitary towels, slippers, dressing gown, deodorant, toiletries, clothes for you

to go home in, flannel, baby wipes, tissues, mobile phone and charger, make up
- *For him*: Su Doku/crossword/ipod/book/nerves of steel
Also don't forget:
- Drinks and snacks
- Ice cubes in a thermos flask to suck between contractions (is anyone this organized?!)
- Unscented oil for massage
- Socks
- A warm fleece
- Spare batteries for TENS machine
- Camera and batteries

Hospital bag aside, the only thing you really need to do in between stopping work and going into labour is rest. You may find that the baby has other ideas, and every time you lie down for some peace and quiet it starts hiccuping, doing the mambo, or sticking its foot into your rib cage. But at least it doesn't make any noise yet.

For great reviews on all baby products, written by mums, visit http://www.mumsnet.com

Baby carriers

Many independent shops offer cheaper versions than the ones below; Mothercare have their own range, and it's worth looking on e-bay (http://www.ebay.co.uk) for second hand ones at good prices.
- Baby Björn: about £50–70 for the standard new born to 1 year carrier, http://www.babybjorn.co.uk
- Bushbaby cocoon: newborn to 4 years, prices from £50 to £180, 0161 474 7097, http://www.bush-baby.com
- Wilkinet Baby Carrier: can be worn on the front or the back, prices start around £42, 01239 841844, http://www.wilkinet.co.uk

References

National Childbirth Trust (September 2004) *Bumps and Babies*, Vol. 1, No. 12. National Childbirth Trust, London.

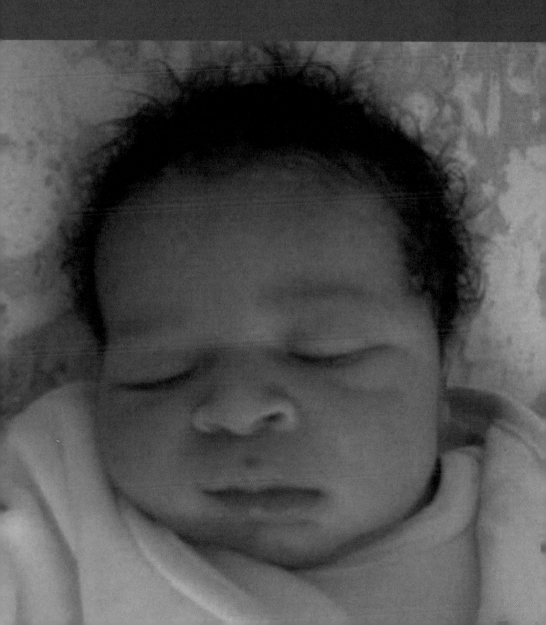

Chapter 10

Doctors giving birth

> In spite of it being a first pregnancy, by the time I reached hospital I was almost fully [dilated] ... It was my brother's wedding day, I was occupied, and I was ignoring my pain ... I kept thinking it was heartburn or something ... Then I realised it was labour pains and I needed to go to the hospital but it was a bit late...

ST obs and gynae

Childbirth is amazing, but as doctors, we've seen things go both ways. Even if your only experience of obstetrics was 15 years ago as a medical student, you'll no doubt have some gruesome dinner party stories. We know that the doctor on the ward might have been a foundation doctor in nuclear medicine until the previous week, and we know that the senior members of the team are probably in theatre or in clinic. We know how the junior doctor must be feeling when they stare blankly at the CTG tracing, then mumble something about phoning their reg. We know that the labour ward is short-staffed with midwives, and that some of the people dealing with you might be temporary staff, new to the team.

> I chose not to have him at X hospital, because having been a registrar there, the only time you got called to labour ward was when there was a disaster, so I sort of associated that with that hospital, and I went to [another] hospital to have my baby.

Consultant physician

Having a medical student present can leave you in a cold sweat as you suddenly remember the teaching session you gave them last year, and now you're grunting and naked, and shouting about vasectomies. You know that deep down they'd rather be at the pub (unless you're pushing as you enter labour ward, in which case they'll be delighted and probably ask you to sign their book while you're being stitched up). When I was a student, we knew that some midwives didn't like us being there, and who could blame them when we rushed in just as the baby was coming out? You may have been left with a residual fear of them. You also probably remember that labour wards can feel unclean, and that emergencies can turn into fumbling disasters if the right person isn't there at the right time. Now is the time to wipe all that from your brain. You are no longer the medical student, you are the patient, and everyone will be doing their best to help you. If you are having the baby in the Trust where you are employed, it is probably quite reasonable to request that no medical students be present if you have teaching duties. If you do have a student present, try and remember how annoying it is for you to give birth after 24 hours of labour, just as they've nipped out for a cup of tea. Aside from all that, you may be having a home birth, or you may be installed at the Portland with a nice glass of Veuve Cliquot.

> I really wanted to have a home birth, we had all the water ready, but I started to get really anxious ... I started to worry about why my labour

was taking so long, and I worried about what was happening to the baby … Then my blood pressure started going up … You almost know too much, being medical, it makes you think the worst …'

Medical student

I suppose that I was quite pushy [on labour ward], saying well I'm not having this and I'm not having that … I'd done lots of obs and gynae, and all the ante natal care here at the practice … And then the most amazing thing was, the consultant came in to theatre, at two o' clock in the morning … Was that because I'm a doctor?! … And [my baby], when he was born, was completely flat, had to be rushed off to be resuscitated, but the SHO forget to label the bloods … I then had the neonatal consultant apologising profusely about the bloods incident, saying 'Oh god, you're a GP, I'm so embarrassed!'

GP

I can't think of anything more terrifying as a junior doctor than having to deal with a consultant or GP patient, especially in an emergency situation, with their medical partner present. The reassuring comments we might try to use with other patients, the stalling techniques while we desperately wait for the registrar to answer their bleep, will all fall on deaf ears. They'll know that 'I just need to show this to my reg,' means we haven't got a clue, and that 'She'll be here in just a minute' is ridiculous if the consultant is gowned up in theatre. So spare a thought for the sweating FY doctor on their fifth attempt at a venflon, or the anaesthetist on their first day at work as a registrar.

The registrar was called for an epidural, and as soon as he saw it was me, he said 'Oh no, I'm going to get the consultant …' but the consultant was at home in his bed! So it took me a lot longer to get the epidural than if the registrar had just done it himself …

Consultant surgeon

My birth turned out to be quite a social event; people I knew kept coming in! First there was the anaesthetist, who was someone I had done research with; but he panicked, and called his consultant in … Then the obstetric consultant came in, whom [my husband] knew, from somewhere he'd worked …

Consultant physician

Better the devil you know?

Pros and cons of having your baby in the hospital you work at (or where you're known as a local GP).

Positive points:

- you might know the obstetric team
- you may not have to wait hours in antenatal clinic; you might be able to nip in and out for your appointment whilst you're working
- you might, if you want it, have consultant care
- your colleagues can come and visit you with chocolates and flowers once you've had the baby
- if things go wrong, you might (rightly or wrongly) have a better chance of receiving optimum care
- you probably won't have to wait too long for your TTA on the day you want to go home

Negative points:

- you might know the obstetric team
- you might not want your colleagues to see you in labour
- your medical students might see you naked
- if you have a difficult delivery, it might taint your view of the hospital, and returning to work afterwards could be difficult
- you might end up with a very 'medicalized' delivery

I had pre-eclampsia and I was in ITU where I worked ... It was fine actually, but I knew most of the staff, I knew most of the anaesthetists. I had a caesarian section at 33 weeks. I did have some extra attention I suppose, the consultant paediatrician came to see me to explain what was going on, then the consultant anaesthetist was going to do my epidural ... But I was mortified, because I knew I would have to be catheterized and have PR voltarol, and I was devastated that all these people who knew me would be doing it... So I sweet talked the nurses into putting the catheter in, on the day of [the section], so the doctors wouldn't do it. Then afterwards, I was looking at my drug chart as only a doctor does, and I saw that I'd been given PR voltarol, and I was mortified! There was me, trying not to expose myself any more than I needed to, and they'd given me PR voltarol

Consultant physician

If you've worked at your hospital for years, or been a local GP for a long time, most senior doctors will either know you, or will know your colleagues. As a result, you might find that people are bending over backwards to help you, and you won't be left with the junior doctor or the student midwife. This may suit you perfectly, or you might feel that your delivery has been 'taken over' and become very medicalized, with all hopes of your water birth fading into the distance.

> To be fair, I was treated very well ... My antenatal care was with a consultant obstetrician who my husband knew vaguely ... The only thing that wasn't done by a consultant in my entire pregnancy was my epidural, when I was in labour. I had to have a caesarian, and the professor of paediatrics was in theatre, waiting for [the baby].
>
> *Consultant physician*

> The consultant said I was going to have a caesarian, he'd popped in lots of times, and been off and done his private list and stuff, and come back, and I was still in labour ... I said 'Listen pal, you talked me out of an elective section a few weeks ago, and if you think I've gone through all this just to have a caesarian, you can think again!
>
> *Consultant surgeon*

Always write a birth plan in your notes. Whether you want a very medicalized birth or not, it gives the staff some idea of what you were hoping for, and stops them assuming that you want every medical intervention possible just because you're a doctor.

> There's one guy, at X hospital, who does all the paediatricians deliveries ... But we can't look him in the eye when we're out socially and we bump into him!
>
> *ST paediatrics*

> I had my second child in the birth centre; I work in the medical obstetric dept, and I chose the consultant I worked with to look after me during pregnancy ... But I wanted to de-medicalize it as much as possible ... It was all absolutely super. I think my colleagues were surprised that I chose the midwife lead centre, but none of them actually said anything to me!
>
> *Consultant diabetologist*

Home births

The current rate of home births in the UK is only about 2%, probably due to a combination of financial constraints, lack of staff, and beliefs about maternity care. The Royal College of Midwives and the Royal College of Obstetricians and Gynaecologists support home births for women who have uncomplicated pregnancies. If you are at low risk of complications, then there is no reason why you should not have the option of delivering your baby at home; it may actually give considerable benefits to you and your family.

If you want to have a home birth, talk to your GP or midwife to discuss the possibility and the options available in your area. You can hire birthing pools for use in your own home if you want a water birth.

Reference: Royal College of Obstetricians and Gynaecologists/Royal College of Midwives Joint statement No. 2, April 2007.

The following day, a midwife came in, she said 'Look, I've come to counsel you,' and I said 'Oh, why? What for?' and she said 'Because your birth was so medicalized ...' And I said 'Oh, no, that's fine, I like medical! I like machines that go ping!' I mean yes, we'd had fetal scalp electrodes, the works ... She said '... But your birth plan ...' and I said 'Oh, s*d the birth plan, I've got a nice, healthy baby!

Consultant surgeon

Not only is it a unique experience to be a doctor and to be a patient, try and sympathize with your partner, if they are there to look after you. If they are a doctor, they might feel totally out of control as they are not in charge; especially if they are more senior than the doctors dealing with you. If your 'birthing partner' is not a doctor, you must make a small pact before you go into labour, namely that you will not be a doctor during the birth. You'll probably struggle to remember your own name, let alone make clinical decisions, so you will have to rely on the people around you, who are there to make the decisions with both of you. This is, by the way, virtually impossible.

My husband [a paediatric surgeon] was single handed at the time, because his colleague was ill, and when I was in labour he was on the phone discussing an exomphalos that was coming in, while I was in labour, obstructed, and that was galling. They managed to stall it [his operation] in the end, so he was there when she was born, but then he had to go and deal with this exomphalos.

Consultant physician

My friend, whose husband was doing his exit exams in surgery, she went into labour on the day of his exam ... And they were sitting with her husband umming and ahing about whether to take her down to theatre ... So they decided let's try to get it out vaginally before he has to go for his exam ... Then he was away for a couple of days when his son was born because he was doing other exams.

ST surgery

You might find, at the other end of the spectrum, that people assume you know what you're doing, and leave you to it. Whether it's because they are intimidated, nervous, or simply don't think you want the 'normal' kind of help, doctors as patients can sometimes feel left out on the ward, with the staff thinking they have no reason to offer them help.

I was a doctor, so they put me in a side room on a completely separate ward, which initially seemed amazing; labour ward was horrible, full of screaming babies, with no privacy and not enough staff. It was great until my husband had gone home, and I had a post partum haemorrhage; because they weren't used to post-natal patients being on the ward, nobody came to do my obs, nobody checked on me.

FY2 doctor

Even if you end up in a private room being waited on hand and foot, you can guarantee that having a baby in hospital will give you a sense of what it is like to be a patient. Some women have never been in hospital for anything else, and suddenly you're on the other side of the fence, wondering why it takes 2 hours to fetch a bed pan when you're desperate for the loo, and what it feels like to be at the sharp end of a tired registrar. For most medics, I think this can only be a positive experience. As doctors, we spend years of our training in hospitals, yet we have no idea what it feels like to be at the mercy of the staff. Being woken up after 2 hours of precious sleep because you have to fill in a menu card; being told off because your husband stayed 10 minutes after visiting time was over; and having people constantly bang the metal bin in your room, usually just after the baby's fallen asleep. You have no idea what patients have to put up with until you're one yourself.

The ward round is some sort of ceremony, and you wait forever for your turn; then, just as you nip to the loo, they come to see you. One glance at the obs chart, and that's it; you ask the nurses whether they want to see you, when you're actually there, as you have some questions. But they're too important for that kind of thing, they haven't got time. In terms of improving my practice, being a patient was the most significant event in my training.

When I was an inpatient, it taught me a lot; the doctors just seemed the most ridiculous people on the ward round ... They'd stand at the end of the bed, and shuffle through a few sheets of paper, and they don't seem very important ... The important people, they were the people who cleaned your room, or who brought you your tea and soup ...

Consultant physician

Some medical students came, who were doing paeds and needed to do their new baby check ... So they took all the clothes off the baby, then their crash bleep went off ... So they said 'Oh we've got to go now, do you mind if we go?' and I said 'Well, would you mind dressing the baby before you go?!'

Consultant physician

Chapter 11

Early days … Yes, it was a baby (not flatus or fluid)

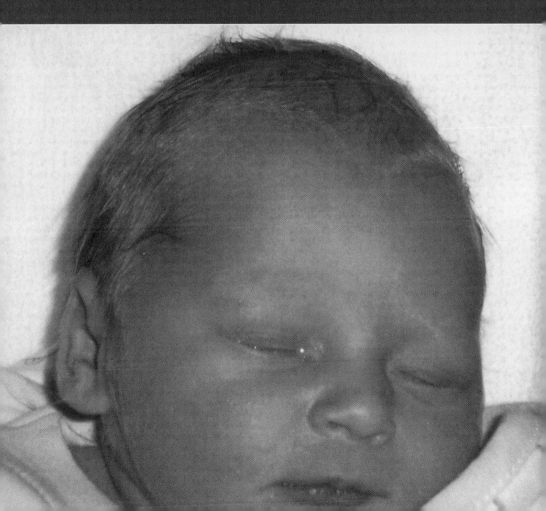

I think some people were really good … But some midwives were almost intimidated … They would say 'Oh ok, you're a medical student, so you know all about it,' but I didn't, I didn't know at all, and I wanted to be told everything, I just wanted to be treated like everyone else … It was a bit frustrating, and anxiety provoking … And I sometimes wouldn't realize I didn't have all the information until after I had left the clinic, then it was too late.

Medical student

Your community midwives and health visitors: Who are they?

Your community midwife will normally visit you at home the day after you leave the hospital. If you have a home birth, you'll know them anyway. They look after you and the baby once you are home, then hand over your care to a Health Visitor between 10 and 28 days after the birth. They are usually brilliant, and can help with everything from breastfeeding to bathing. They'll also give you a contact number, so you can ring if you're worried about anything. Mine was absolutely fantastic, as her first words to me were 'Right, I know what you doctors are like, you listen to me and do what I say.' It was definitely the correct approach, and even now she pops in for a cup of tea if she's visiting someone nearby.

I remember the community midwives being brilliant, and not treating me like a doctor, they gave me all sorts of brilliant tips.

GP

Health Visitors are qualified nurses, who have received extra training in looking after people in the community. Their main interest is in the health of the family, especially those with very young children; they'll be able to advise you on problems with feeding and sleeping, behavioural issues, and are there to help if you're having problems coping.

Whatever you do, don't waddle round the house with an ice pack on your backside trying to tidy up or do the hoovering before they arrive. They will not call social services because your house is in chaos. Their job is to visit new mums.

I felt that I didn't know anything about [babies] anyhow, and so I wasn't expecting to know what to do … You really have to depend on other people.

Consultant physician

The midwives on the ward didn't know what cup feeding was … I'd cup fed on a neonatal unit, so I showed them how to do it!

ST paediatrics

Postnatal check for you (not the baby)

This is supposed to happen 6–8 weeks after the birth, but not all surgeries will tell you, so make sure you call and make an appointment if they don't contact you. Despite being tempted to do our own postnatal checks, or phone a friend, it's probably best to get the GP or midwife to do it; it's to make sure that you're ok physically and emotionally, and they'll want to do things such as take your blood pressure, check if you have any discharge, check the size of your uterus, and examine your perineum if you had stitches and/or tears. They should ask about contraception, even though you may feel more like chopping your own head off than having sex.

Having sex after childbirth

I remember being told as a medical student that people were often caught 'doing it' on the postnatal wards. I suspect that either this was a lie, or that those people were mad. If you want to have sex, you are apparently meant to wait for about 6 weeks. If your breasts explode every time you move, and you are completely sleep deprived and exhausted, don't worry. Remember that everything gets back to normal eventually. Something that even doctors can forget is that you can get pregnant straight away, even if you are exclusively breastfeeding. If that's not enough to put you off, I don't know what is.

What on earth is the baby clinic?

Your health visitor will tell you when to go—the first visit is usually to weigh the baby, and see the health visitor on site.

The baby clinic gives you a chance to meet with other new mums, and to see the health visitor, and often the GP if you need to. Your baby will also be weighed. Although the prospect may seem very daunting, it can be a very reassuring time too; you realize that you're not the only one to have forgotten nappies/a cloth for the baby's vomit/spare clothes, and it may be the first time you breastfeed 'in public,' and it's a nice environment to do that in.

Some surgeries have a special room set aside for baby clinic; others expect you all to pile into the waiting room with everyone else. Bear in mind that if you can take your baby in a sling, it's probably easier than taking the pram, as some surgeries may not have enough space, and you may need to leave your pram outside.

Take a bottle of water and snacks for you, and spare nappies, clothes, and bottles if needed for the baby. Wearing breast pads may help, as you may be called in to see two or three different people, and have to interrupt your baby's feeding several times.

You'll feel terrible if you forget to take the Red Book along, which is your child's personal health record. Don't be 'That doctor that forgot their book.'

Immunization schedules: what everybody will expect you to know

- **6 weeks**: BCG in certain areas—one injection
- **2 months**: diphtheria, tetanus, pertussis, polio and *Haemophilus influenza* type B (DTaP, IPV, Hib)—one injection
- **3 months**: pneumococcal vaccine (PCV), one injection; DTaP, IPV, Hib, one injection—plus Meningitis C (MenC), one injection, i.e. three jabs
- **4 months**: PCV, one injection; DTaP, IPV, Hib, one injection—plus MenC, one injection, i.e. three jabs
- **12 months**: Hib and Men C, one injection
- **13 months**: measles, mumps and rubella (MMR), one injection
- **Pre-school (at approximately age 3 and a half to 5)**: diphtheria, tetanus, pertussis and polio, one injection—plus MMR, one injection
- **Age 13–18 years**: diphtheria, tetanus, and polio, one injection
- Check http://www.immunisation.nhs.uk for the most up-to-date information

Some women struggle in more ways than one after the birth of a baby. It has long been known that women who have given birth have a higher rate of mental illness following the event; it is also well known that if untreated, perinatal psychiatric disorders can prolong maternal morbidity, as well as interfering with bonding (Kannabiran *et al.* 2007). It can feel incredibly lonely at times, stuck in the house with a baby who seems to cry all the time, but remember that there are plenty of places to look for help; your health visitor, community midwife, and GP will all be looking out for signs of postnatal problems, and will be able to help.

Postnatal depression and baby blues

The Scottish Intercollegiate Guidelines Network-60 (SIGN 60): http://www.sign.ac.uk/pdf/sign60.pdf

Postnatal blues/baby blues:
This is described as a brief episode that can affect about half of all women after delivery, of tearfulness and feeling miserable. It is more common with first babies.

Postnatal depression
This occurs in 10–15% of women after childbirth. It includes any non-psychotic depressive illness during the first year after the birth of the baby. It is described as being of mild to moderate severity.

However many births you've been present at, seeing your baby for the first time is a whole new experience. Whether you're overcome with maternal love or too stunned to think straight, over the next few days it will start to sink in that you're finally a mum; congratulations!

There comes a day in every new mum's life when you are sent home to cope with your first baby. If you had a home birth you will, of course, already be there. You may have two degrees, a doctorate, a host of publications, and a place on several committees, but you now have to deal with a very small person who seems upset a lot of the time, and who doesn't care how clever you are. Some women have their mum to help them, others have sisters or a mother in law, or friends, but some have to cope on their own, with or without the baby's father.

This should be a wonderful time in your life, but it is also a time when you can feel isolated and cut off from you family and friends, weary from lack of sleep, and at a loss to knowing what your role is, having previously been a professional woman in a position of some importance. It is normal for new mums to have bad days, or even bad weeks, but the important thing is to seek help before things start to spiral out of control.

> I didn't know anyone here [I had had an interdeanery transfer because my husband had changed jobs], and I actually had postnatal depression ... My health visitor was very supportive, and she put me in touch with other mums who had similar problems ... And I did a few parenting courses, FamilyLinks, which really helped. The older child didn't like the baby, she was two and a half, and she regressed a bit, with her toileting and everything. I found it all really hard ... I caught her one day; she'd climbed on top of the carry cot, and was lying right on top of the baby ... It all seemed out of control, the place was a complete tip, and I was wandering around in my dressing gown at lunchtime, just chaos ... I remember the health visitor coming round, and I had completely forgotten ... But I used to be so organized ... But a few months later, things settled down.
>
> *Consultant physician*

'Early Days' is a booklet produced by the National Childbirth Trust (NCT), full of helpful advice to enjoy the first few weeks with your baby. It costs £2.50 plus 50p P&P, just call the NCT on 0870 112 1120.

I actually had postnatal depression both times. Nobody seemed to recognize it, but I felt that I was screaming out … I was cracking up, but I could put on a good face … It was only when it was all over; my husband said 'Oh, you're back!' I had a lot of support from the Health Visitor and the GP, but nobody wanted to label it … It took about nine months to go … So everyone was on red alert the second time, but I thought well, I know what to look for, and this time I've got my friends, my family … But it was horrible, it hit again, and I recognized it. I had to be persuaded to go on to antidepressants, I even phoned up the manufacturers of one of the drugs, such a typical doctor! But actually, taking them was the best thing I ever did.

Consultant surgeon

Registering your baby's birth

England and Wales

It is a legal requirement to register the birth within 42 days, at your local register office (look online or in the phone book for your nearest office). This sounds like a long time, but if you're still arguing about the name, it can fly by.

The Registrar will need to know the sex of the baby, and the place and time of birth. If you are married, then either you or your husband can register the birth; if you aren't married, you are not obliged to provide the father's details, but it's wise to put his name on the certificate if you want him to share responsibilities. The hospital (or midwife) should issue you with a document with the baby's hospital registration number on it.

The Registrar needs your full names, surnames, and dates and places of your births. They also need your address, and your occupations. If you are married, then you need to know the date of your marriage, and as the mum you'll need to inform them of any previous children you may have had from this marriage, and from any previous marriage.

The Registrar will give you a free (short) birth certificate, which you will need in order to claim your child benefit. They will also issue you with a form to take to your GP, in order to register the baby there. For a small fee, you can have a longer form of the certificate. At this point, it's probably sensible to ask for a couple of spare copies; they cost a few pounds each.

Scotland and Northern Ireland

In Scotland you only have 21 days to register the birth; in Northern Ireland you have 42 days.

I started my first job on 1st august, full-time, when he was only three and a half weeks old … It's a bit of a blur now!

FY1 doctor

Being a doctor and being a new mum

If you thought that your self-diagnosis skills were a bit rusty, just wait until you have a new baby to diagnose. If you have a high threshold for taking your baby to the GP surgery, because you've seen thousands of kids with viral diarrhoea and vomiting, and you know what to do, the other mums around you might wonder if you're a complete witch. On the other hand, you can have a sudden panic that something might be seriously wrong, and you've just been 'watching and waiting' for days, in which case you end up feeling guilty.

I seem to fluctuate between compete paranoia and total negligence with my children …. I never know whether I'm doing the right thing.

GP

Doctors are apparently supposed to know what to do and to do all the right things, so eyebrows might be raised if you wean them too early or too late, if you don't breast-feed, and if you drive round the block five hundred times a day just to get the baby to sleep. The reality is that we are just like any other new mums, and have to learn by trial and error, and we can't be perfect. You will know what's best for your baby, so the only thing to do is ignore any 'helpful advice' you feel you don't need.

For god's sake, don't buy any baby books … One tells you to do this, another one tells you to do that … I ended up feeling completely stressed out and depressed, confused, and I felt like I wasn't doing anything right. My husband made me chuck them all away … Just do what feels right.

ST medicine

Some doctors decide to invent a parallel life so they don't have to confess to being medically trained. It can start at the antenatal classes, while you're struggling to remember how many stages of labour there are ('we've got a doctor here, if anyone's got any questions?'). It may continue with the health visitor, who thinks you know how to cope when you can't even work out how to do up the poppers on the babygro. It can even transcend into the GP consultation: 'So, have you listened to her chest yourself?' Not even in my wildest dreams would I try to examine my own baby properly, for fear of diagnosing bilateral pneumonia and congenital cardiac disease, resulting in a frantic rush to A&E with my long-suffering husband in tow. Not only would I be incompetent, but my stethoscope has reached into the groins of obese vascular patients to listen for bruits, and even one hundred sterets later still feels tainted.

It's really quite simple; when your baby is unwell, see your GP, or take them to A&E if it's serious, like any normal non-doctor would. This usually only dawns on me after I've left several messages on friends' voicemails, asking for advice, and bleeped friends away from their consultant ward rounds. Being a mum for your baby is quite enough to cope with, so don't think you have to be their doctor too.

The other difficult thing about the very early days is keeping in touch with your friends who are working full time. They often call in the evenings after work, when your baby has finally gone to sleep for a short while, and you are trying to wolf down some dinner. Or you may be busy breastfeeding and trying to eat at the same time. You probably feel desperate to talk to people in the daytime, when you're stuck on the sofa in the middle of a two hour breastfeeding marathon, and the remote control's broken with the television stuck on Bargain Hunt. These are the times when you'll be able to turn to any new friends you've made, who have also had babies, and who also feel lonely during the day. Just remember, if you're having a bad day, this phase doesn't last forever! Before you know it, your baby will be a crawling, stumbling, babbling toddler, and you'll wonder how on earth it happened so quickly. You and your baby are both learning about each other, and becoming entwined in each others feelings and emotions, and without even trying you'll be falling in love.

References

Kannabiran M, Narayan G (2007) Perinatal psychiatry. *BMJ Career Focus* **334**: 75–76.

Royal College of General Practitioners (Autumn/Winter 2004/5) *Emma's Diary*. Royal College of General Practitioners, London. http://www.emmasdiary.co.uk/postnatal/postnatal_body.html

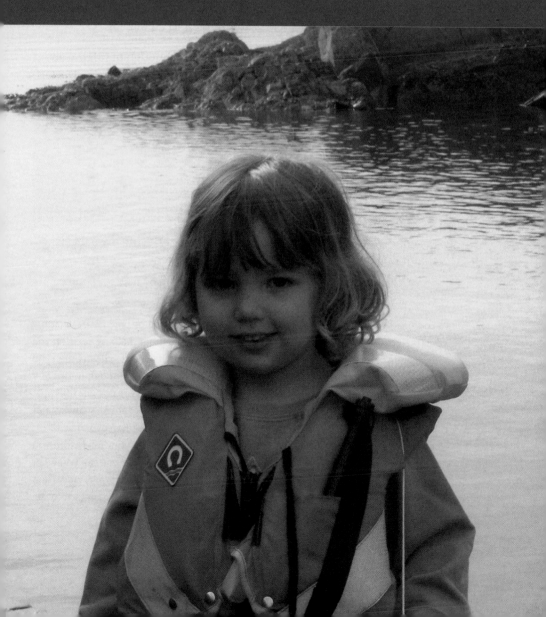

Planning your return to work

ı had a real battle with myself, whether to take out six months or a year … In the end I decided to take a year. It seems such a big deal but it's only a year! You can never get that time [with your baby] back … And you'll always be working; even when your children are older, you'll still be working. You're going to be working for another 30 years, what's the big deal about 12 months?

ST general practice

For the first part of your maternity leave, you can push any thought of your 'proper' job to the back of your mind and forget about it. But there will come a time, sooner or later, when you will either want to go back, or have to go back for financial reasons. It shouldn't be all doom and gloom though—as I mentioned at the start of this book, we have a great career that we worked hard for, so if you want to go back, don't feel guilty! You are a mother, and nobody can take that away from you, but you are also a doctor, and getting back to your role at work can be a very rewarding.

I was really ready to go back to work … I'd had enough of talking about breastfeeding. I'd applied to be a flexible trainee in fact while I was off, but it wasn't until three weeks before I had to go back that I knew I had a flexible post! It wasn't straightforward [to organize], and there was a lot of wrangling about the on calls …

Consultant physician

If you are unwell and unable to return to work following the end of your maternity leave, normal sick leave provisions apply.

My concern about taking a whole year off [after having my baby] is that it might be quite hard to go back … Confidence-wise and everything.

Medical student

You need to decide how you are going to work, full time or part time. Deciding what is right for you and your family is difficult, but remember that any decision you make needn't be set in stone. If you go back part time, and it doesn't suit you, then you can always apply to return to full-time work (as long as you give enough notice and there is a post available). If you can't get a part-time job, and have to go back full time, it shouldn't be for ever, and with perseverance you might get what you want sooner than you think. Some women decide not to go back to work, or take several years off to be with their family. A lot will depend on how you felt about your job before you got pregnant, and how far you are through your training. Nobody can tell you what to do, and what is right for one family will be wrong for another. If you're uncertain about what to do, your consultant, consultant colleagues, or partners may be extremely helpful to talk to, and may be able to put you in touch with other doctors who had doubts about returning to work. Remember that if you can't stand the thought of going back to work and leaving your baby, you may feel differently in a year's time; don't spend all your early days with the baby worrying about it.

> The mistake that I see most girls make, and I tell them, is that nought to five years old is your time … The children don't really notice a lot if you're there or not … You think that as they get older, they'll demand less time and energy, but actually they need more … So don't think 'Well, I'll put it all on hold until they're five…' I've seen a few women make that mistake, they think 'Well, I'll get all my time with them when they're little, then I'll go full time,' but it doesn't work like that.'
>
> *Consultant colo-rectal surgeon*

Full-time work

Many doctors go back full time after their maternity leave; for some, it's the only option financially, and for others there may not be the opportunity for part-time work. Many women go back full time because they enjoy their jobs, and don't feel that they can work in the way they want to in a part-time capacity. Going back full time can be a real shock to the system at first, and you need to have a lot of faith in your childcare, but if it works for you, it means that you get to progress more quickly in your chosen field.

> I planned to take off three months, but because he was prem I took off five months and went back full time … My boss persuaded me to do a care of the elderly rehab job, but I wanted to go for cardiology or something, I thought there's no way I'm doing rehab, I'm a career doctor! But the on calls were quiet, and actually it was the right thing to do.
>
> *Consultant physician*

> It's not worth being a part time consultant … You only work five days a week anyway and the weekends are ok … The pay is so much less part time and you still have to do the same amount of work, just in less time … The children are at school, so I leave at 8am, then the children leave at quarter past 8. They get home at four then I'm home by half six, they've either got a friend round, or football, or TV, then I get home and can play, or help with projects.
>
> *Consultant physician*

Remember that before you had the baby, you could go in early and stay late; the only person who missed you was the cat, or your partner (although he was probably working late too). Little babies sleep at the strangest times, and not much at night, but toddlers may sleep from 7 p.m. to 7 a.m., i.e. the only time you're at home. Don't underestimate the emotional drain of working full time, as well as the physical one. If you're having problems coping, then try and find other doctors who have been through a similar experience. Try and remember that little babies are happy being with anyone who loves them, and they won't remember the early days once they've grown up!

> I went back to work full time partly for money, but also I didn't want to be juggling the baby and my partner working as well ... There was the option, but I'd spoken to people who'd worked part time, and they don't feel part of the team.. They felt they didn't know the patients. Being full time has been fine, I'm really enjoying all sides of life!

FY1 doctor

Part time work

> These part-time doctors ... I don't know what they think they need all the time off for ... Shopping I suppose.

Male consultant cardiologist

You will need to work at least 50% of the working week. If full-time trainees in your speciality have Out of Hours (OOH) commitments, you will be expected to complete the relevant percentage of OOH (but you are allowed a 6-month period without OOH for exceptional circumstances). You are not allowed to take on any other paid employment, including locum work.

Your salary will, of course, be less once you work part time. Hospital doctors need to be aware that working at 60% does not necessarily mean that you will earn 60% of your full-time salary. If you are doing a supernumerary post, as a junior hospital doctor, your Trust may or may not be able to fund OOH. If they can't, then your salary will be 60% of basic salary (giving you a gross of maybe £15 000). If you are on a job share at 80%, your Trust will probably only allow you to work 50% of your OOH (as they don't see the need to pay two people to be on call together), so your gross salary will be 80% of basic, plus pay for only half of the OOH commitment. OOH banding makes a significant part of hospital doctors pay, so make sure you do your sums before you commit to part-time work.

Table 12.1. Converting full time to part time equivalents

	12 months full time	24 months full time	36 months full time
At 50%	2 years	4 years	6 years
At 60%	20 months	40 months	60 months
At 70%	17 months	34 months	51 months
At 80%	15 months	30 months	45 months

Your total salary will be made up of two elements:

1. *Basic salary band* (based on the number of actual hours you work per week). This is then calculated as a proportion of your full-time basic salary:

   - Band F5 (you work 20–24 hours per week) you earn 0.5 of your basic salary
   - Band F6 (you work 24–28 hours per week) you earn 0.6 of your basic salary
   - And so on, up to Band F9 (36–40 hours, 0.9 of your basic salary).

2. *Intensity supplement*. This is only payable if you work antisocial hours. If you work less than 40 hours a week in total, and these fall between 8 a.m. and 7 p.m., Monday to Friday, then you are not eligible for an intensity supplement.

   - FA: working at high intensity, and at the most antisocial hours—50%
   - FB: working at less intensity, at less antisocial times—40%
   - FC: duties outside the period 8 a.m. to 7 p.m., Monday to Friday—20%

     The percentage is the supplement payable as a proportion of the calculated basic salary.

As an ST3 in General Practice, your pay will be calculated in a different way. You will be paid on a pro rata basis compared with your full-time colleagues.

People who call part-time working 'half time' ... Well, I used to think 'Look, I've never seen you racing around Tesco's at eleven o clock at night ...'

Consultant surgeon

Types of training post:

1. Slot share: one training job is split between two trainees. You are employed and paid as individuals, usually at 60%.
2. Supernumerary post: these posts are additional to the usual numbers of staff members on the rota.
3. Job share: a full-time post is shared by two trainees. Each doctor gets half the salary, and works half the hours.

In order to be approved for flexible training, you need a 'well founded individual reason.' Category 1 applicants are considered first; people with a disability or ill health, caring responsibility for a child or children, caring for a relative, parent or dependant who is ill or disabled. Category 2 includes doctors who are, for example, training to compete nationally or internationally in a sport, who have religious commitments, or who wish to develop non-medical interests such as law or fine art courses. Category 1 applicants are prioritized by the deanery. Flexible training contracts are usually approved for 1 year at a time.

> If you want to increase or decrease your sessions, you need to make sure you give plenty of notice; this can, if it is accepted, take several months.

I'm going back as a job share, because in our department they've changed the rules on part time working as a supernumerary doctor ... They restricted the supernumerary slots to four, so once they were all taken up; people couldn't come back part time, even if they had kids ... So it was decided that was a bit unfair and we can job share, doing three days a week each ... It's easy to do a job share in radiology, because your work is based around a morning and an afternoon list, you're sort of sharing, but it's easier [than sharing ward work.]

ST radiology

If you do a job share with someone, you need to make sure that you get on well at a personal level, and can communicate easily with each other. You'll probably have one day, or one session, overlapping, where you can do a proper handover. If one of you always works Monday, Tuesday, and Wednesday, and the other works Wednesday, Thursday, and Friday, then you might find that one or the other of you misses out on certain meetings and experiences. If you can organize your childcare, you can try and swap around half way through the post, in order to make sure that neither of you misses out.

A summary of the application process:

1. Talk to the postgraduate dean for flexible training to seek advice on eligibility.
2. Apply to train flexibly. In other words, you need to apply for a full-time post in open competition. You do not have to state your intention to train flexibly at interview, or on the application form.
3. Agree your training programme with your deanery.
4. The training programme must now be approved by the regional speciality education committee or programme director, and the postgraduate deanery.

Being a part-time doctor: pros and cons

Positive points:

- You get to spend more time with your children
- You may appreciate your time at work more, as you're not wishing you were at home

- If you are supernumerary, you should be welcomed by the rest of the team as an extra person
- If you're an extra person, you can probably leave on time most days, and if you or your children are sick, there's less of an impact if you're not there
- If you're supernumerary, you can probably take your annual leave whenever you want it.

Negative points:

- Your pay will drop dramatically (especially if you can't get funding for OOH)
- Hospital doctors may feel that they can't keep up with what's happening to patients on the ward
- You may not feel part of the team
- Your training will take longer to complete
- You may feel that you're not fulfilling your potential as a doctor
- As a supernumerary doctor, you can sometimes feel as if you're a medical student, an extra person; it's not that great if nobody notices you were off on sick leave!

As a GP, working part-time will probably be seen as a more 'normal' thing to do; working less than 10 sessions a week will not be perceived as a strange thing to do. In some specialities, you may find that you are unusual.

I went back three days a week. The SHOs who were there were highly demoralized, and they were forever moaning … And I'd got a life outside work, which I think they begrudged me … And they would divvy up all the jobs and just give me something to do, but I felt like, well where's my role in all this? I think it's harder being part time the more junior you are … You pitch up, and when you're the reg, the SHOs will fill you in and tell you what's happening … When you're an SHO you just have to muck in … It was horrible, when the consultants came on the ward on a Tuesday and asked what was going on, and I hadn't been there on the Monday, I felt useless, terrible … But when I was a registrar it was easier.

Consultant physician

I've been a registrar for ever … X, he was my SHO, and now he's applying for consultant jobs … But you know what, I think I've gained so much from taking this long to train; having a family has made me so different. I used to be really headstrong, really fiery, but now I've mellowed, and nothing stresses me! I'm sure if I hadn't [had kids] then I'd have become a consultant really quickly and what have you … But I'm going to be a much better consultant, because I've done things my way.

ST paediatrics

As a part-time doctor, you have to be fairly proactive, depending on how organized your Deanery and HR department is. You might long for the days when you just turned up and got paid, without having to organize your own post, write detailed job descriptions, hassle payroll as they continue to pay you the wrong amount, or not at all, keep a detailed log book of all the work you do, and organize your own inductions and visits to occupational health, etc. (you'll probably start and end posts at different times to everyone else). Each job you do must get approval for your training, and there may be issues sorting out funding. I can't stress this enough; plan your posts well in advance, months in advance, because if you leave it until the last minute you could end up without a job.

I got a phone call on the day the baby was due, from the Deanery, saying [my flexible post] wasn't going to work because I needed to fill in this form and that form … So I rang the woman at the Deanery at this end and said 'Look, I'm meant to be having my baby today, and they're giving me hassle!' I just couldn't believe they were doing it on that day.

Consultant surgeon

Your annual leave will be calculated on a pro rata arrangement. Make sure that your contract states your entitlement in writing. You should not be disadvantaged if you don't work Mondays (i.e. bank holidays); the days of leave that you would have got as a full-time doctor should be calculated by you; talk to HR to check your entitlements. If you are working part time, you will be entitled to both paid and unpaid maternity leave under the NHS scheme, as outlined in Chapter 8.

Food for thought: working six sessions per week

- three whole days
- two days plus two mornings/two afternoons/one of each
- one day plus four mornings
- one day plus four afternoons
- one day plus a mixture of mornings and afternoons

Working **whole days** means you are able to concentrate on your work all day. You get more whole days with your children. There are fewer opportunities to be late to nursery/the childminder's/work. You may feel more of a 'team member' in hospital medicine, as you arrive and leave with the normal day staff.

If your child is unwell on a working day, you miss two sessions. If you are fully breastfeeding and your baby is young it can be hard work (see Chapter 13), but is not impossible. Never underestimate how exhausting a full day can be, with young children at home, especially if they don't sleep through the night.

Working **mornings** means that you can feel like a normal working person, except you get to leave early. If your child has breakfast early, it may mean that you get to be with them for three meals a day. If you are a hospital doctor you may want to be on, or lead, ward rounds that take place in the mornings.

You might feel too exhausted in the afternoons to enjoy your children properly. You can feel that you spend the whole morning rushing around like a headless chicken trying to get everything done at work so you can leave on time. You may feel guilty if you don't go to 'lunchtime teaching' in hospital posts, but these can go on until 1 or 2 p.m. and most nurseries or childminders want you to collect your child by 1 o'clock. Morning surgeries in general practice can run late.

Working **afternoons** mean that you can still spend the best part of the day with your children, when they're not too tired. But it may mean that you spend all morning 'getting ready to go to work' both physically and mentally.

It may be easier to leave on time than if you work mornings, as most people are leaving at the same time as you. It can be difficult tracking everyone down at lunchtimes in hospital, to find out what's going on and what needs doing, and you may find that you miss most of the ward rounds.

He [my partner] got a job miles up north, it took us away from our families and everything, and the baby was only about three months old … I knew I wanted to do renal, but I just thought well, I'll have to try and get in at the back door… That's when I found out about flexible training and supernumerary posts … I rang the consultant nephrologist, and it was the most demeaning telephone call I've ever had; I was trying to tell him how much I wanted to do renal medicine, be enthusiastic, and he cut me short, and said 'Look, do you come free [of cost?]' And when I said yes, he said 'Fine, then we'll have you.' … I felt like oh, right, well that's not made me feel great … I've always worked hard for what I've got, I felt like I was just filling a service need

Consultant renal physician

Flexible training doesn't have to be for ever, if you don't want it to be. One study showed that of all registrars in flexible training jobs, almost half worked part time for less than 3 years, a third for 4–6 years, and less than one-fifth for over 7 years. The study demonstrated that registrars in the UK who trained flexibly were as likely to get their Certificate of Completion of Training, and to take a consultant post in the NHS, as their full-time colleagues.

www.bma.org.uk/ for more information on flexible training, including the annual flexible training forum at BMA House

You do miss out [as a part time doctor] … I've seen everyone overtaking me … Your house officer, suddenly they're your consultant, and you're there saying 'No, I'm a reg, yes still a reg,' and its demoralizing … But I'm incredibly lucky: I've seen my kids grow up, I love my job, and I've got to where I wanted …

Consultant renal physician

Most of the Royal Colleges have an adviser for flexible training. Make sure you talk to the adviser for your speciality early on.

I was working full time when I had my third baby, and I hated it … I think I actually got post-natal depression. I was sick of handing everything over each day, the children and the house, to nannies and cleaners … When I changed to general practice, I went onto the retainer scheme, and I did two mornings a week, then three mornings, for five years. Then, I went onto the flexible careers scheme.

GP

Dealing with negative attitudes from colleagues as a part-time doctor

Hopefully, you won't encounter any. The vast majority of doctors are fascinated, and often envious, of your work–life balance. Occasionally, you can be made to feel like a bit of a second-class doctor, and the following might help:

- Never say 'I'm only part time,' or 'Sorry, I only work part time. Say 'I work part time.'

- If you're a junior ward doctor, and a consultant or registrar from another team is coming to review one of your patients, don't apologize for being part time if you weren't there the previous day; a full time doctor may have been away on annual leave, study leave, or off sick. If you don't know the patient, and don't have a chance to meet them first, simply explain that you weren't on the ward yesterday, and go with the consultant to help them if you can. At the very least, find them the notes and show them where the patient is.

- Lots of people will ask you 'What do you do on your days off?' Remember that before you had kids, you had no idea how busy a day with two young children was; don't huff and puff about it 'not being a day off …' It is fun being with your kids!

- Make sure that you have as much opportunity as your peers for attending courses, going to teaching sessions and meetings. If your name isn't on lists for presentations or case discussions, ask to be added on.

Job splitting

This allows two consultants to apply for a single full-time post and divide them into two part-time posts (Dick and Walker 2007). Each consultant has an independent employment contract. It is different from a job share, as there is less restriction to the programmed activities (PAs) and you don't need to reapply for your job if your partner resigns. To find the perfect partner, you need to:

1. Have similar plans for the next 5 years, in terms of where you want to live.
2. Have similar, or complementary, subspecialty interests.
3. Have similar approaches.
4. Find someone who will interview as well as you, to make sure you both get the job!

Returners scheme for general practice

The [GP] Returners that I work with, they're amazing, a very mixed group of people … Men and women, some who have been off through ill health, others who have had children …. One was a medical journalist, and another has a disabled child who she cares for … It's a great scheme. They need to prove their competence in an MCQ exam, and in a simulated surgery, and if they can get through that, it doesn't matter how long they've had off from clinical work.

GP

The National Returner Scheme was launched by the Department of Health in 2002. It included the introduction of the GP Returner scheme in England, to facilitate a programme of re-entry into general practice by means of refresher training. The GP Returner scheme funded a period of refresher training of 6 months or less, which could be done full time or part time. The scheme was highly successful, and increased the recruitment of GPs; it was especially helpful for women who had taken time off to have children. Ninety-eight doctors were placed on the London Deanery scheme between 2003 and 2006, of whom 65% were female; 67% did the scheme on a part-time basis. The Department of Health withdrew funding for the scheme in 2006, and there is currently no budget for the Deaneries to work with. It's worth noting that in order to practise as an NHS GP in the UK; you must be on the new GMC register and also on a Primary Care Organization's (PCO's) Performers list. You will not be allowed on to the GP performer's list unless you have been working as an NHS GP within the last 2 years.

(The above information was kindly supplied by Naureen Bhatti, course organizer for the GP induction and refresher scheme, London Deanery.)

References

BMA Junior Doctors Committee (2005) A guide to New Deal flexible training. *Junior Doctors Annual Report 2005*. British Medical Association, London.

Dick E, Walker M. (2007) Splitting a consultant job. *BMJ Career Focus* **334**: 108–109.

Gray SF, Goodyear HM, Jones MJT. Outcomes of flexible training compared to full-time training during the specialist registrar grade in the UK (2005). Med Educ online http://www.med-ed-online.org

Pritchard, L. (2007) Ministers wish GPs many unhappy returns. BMA news, March 24 2007.

Chapter 13

Breastfeeding and working

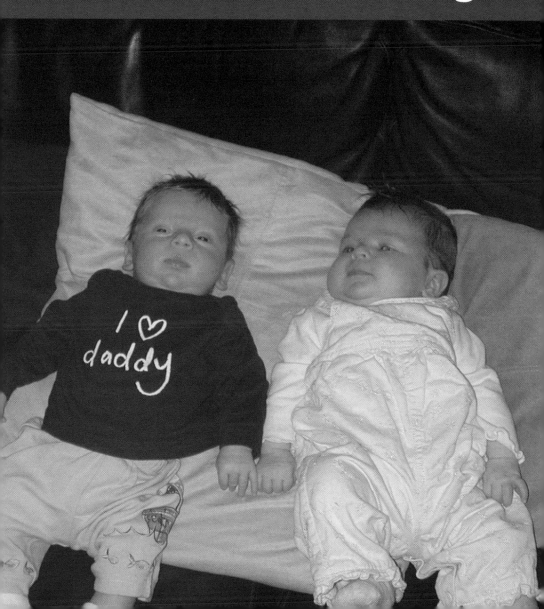

There was a fantastic doctor's mess, and a crèche attached to the hospital, so I would go and drop him off and feed him, then do clinic … The neuro rehab job meant it was all clinics, so the timing was easy, then I could go and have a play and feed him again … So I managed to breastfeed for about a year despite working full time.

Consultant physician

As doctors, we all know that breastfeeding is the best thing for babies, and for mothers too. If you breastfeed your baby, you'll need to decide what you want to do once you return to work. If you want to, you can still breastfeed once you've gone back, but if you can't cope, or don't want to, the main thing to remember is that babies need happy mothers more than they need breast milk.

In practice, there are four main options, as outlined below. A lot will depend upon the age of the baby, and whether they have started eating solids:

1. **The baby has only breast milk.** This is certainly possible, but can be tiring if you are working full-time. You will only have a certain number of hours at home each day, and you need to remember to feed yourself, breastfeed the baby, sleep, *and* express the milk for the next day. You'll also need to sterilize all the expressing equipment, bottles, etc. You may find that you're spending all your time at home with either a baby or a whirring machine attached to you; not a thought to cherish. You'll also need to express during the working day, in order to avoid agony and keep your supply going. If there's a fridge available, you can keep this milk and take it home with you (just make sure it doesn't get used by the ward clerk for her tea). If there's no fridge, then the milk you express at work will probably all have to go to waste.

   Some hospital nurseries will allow you to go and breastfeed your baby during the day. Something to bear in mind is that during the first few months, babies take ages to feed. So unless you're strictly feeding by the clock, or taking the baby off after 10 minutes, it's probably going to take up a fair part of your day.

You can download the Breastfeeding Network leaflet (September 2004) from http://www.breastfeedingnetwork.org.uk/pdfs/BFNExpressing&Storing.pdf for evidence based advice on expressing and storing breast milk

I would get in from uni and then start expressing, time I should have spent with her, I was attached to the pump, desperately trying to get enough milk for the next day. It felt a bit wrong, she would be trying to cuddle me, but I had to concentrate on the stupid machine.

Medical student

2. **You want to breastfeed the baby when you are with them, but they will have formula milk when you're not around.** Lots of people, even medics, may tell you that you can't do this because your milk supply will 'dry up,' making you sound like a desiccated coconut, despite knowing that milk production is a positive feedback mechanism. As long as you keep feeding your baby every day, even if just on waking and at bedtime, your milk supply should keep going. If you're on late shifts, you can take a pump to work and express milk at some point in the evening. If you think you're not producing enough, try the usual things; express more, and feed more when you're with the baby.
3. **You want your baby to have breast milk when they wake up and go to bed, and formula the rest of the time, even when you're with them**.
4. **Your baby has formula and no breast milk.**
   Any combination of the above will probably work; as long as it works for you and the baby, then it's the right thing to do (whatever your family, friends, or colleagues think). You are a busy woman doing a busy job, and being a mother generally gives you enough things to feel guilty about without putting added pressure on yourself.

I breastfed, I think, to make me feel better [when I went back to work]. I'd weaned him during the day, because I couldn't be dealing with expressing and all that, but then I found that quite often, he really didn't want a breast feed first thing in the morning before I went to work, he just wanted to play with his toys and stuff ... So it was just more of a hassle. And the evening feed, well I was just getting home too late. I didn't want her [the nanny] to keep him up, just so I could breastfeed him. I probably breastfed for just two weeks when I went back.

GP

Advice from the Health and Safety Executive

- Provide your employer with written notification that you are breastfeeding, ideally before you return
- Your employer is then obliged to carry out a Risk Assessment (see later)
- Your employer is required by law to provide somewhere for you to 'rest,' but is not required to provide somewhere suitable for expressing (or storing) milk.
- HSE states that a toilet is not a suitable place for expressing milk

My friend used to express at work ... But there don't seem to be any good facilities here, other than the toilet or the on-call room, so I assume that's what everyone else does.

ST anaesthetics

[By the time I had my baby] I had been a GP for six years, and I'd done paediatrics, and advised loads of mums on feeding, breastfeeding ... I really did feel like I knew what to do ... But I don't think you really become an expert until you become a parent

GP

Advice from doctors who have breastfed

- Take a spare top to work. The last thing you want to do is lead a ward round with a tide mark on your shirt.

- Wear breast pads at all times, even if you are tailing off feeding.

- Electric pumps are very noisy, so you may prefer expressing with a hand pump at work

- The 'freezer bag' style sterilizing bags are great, as you can sterilize your equipment quickly and take it in your bag to work the next day without it taking up too much room.

I tried going into the toilets to express ... But it didn't really work out for me. So I went over to the maternity wards, and they were a bit surprised at first, but then they showed me how to use their breast pumps, and after a month or so I was pretty good at it! I used to do my medical registrar on call, sat with a pump on each breast, a phone, a bleep, and a piece of paper, taking calls and directing the on-call ... I used to put my milk in the fridge with my name on it, with the other mum's milk, and take it home in a cool bag.

Consultant physician

National Childbirth Trust Breastfeeding Line

- 0870 444 8708
- 7 days a week from 8 a.m. to 10 p.m.

An excellent source of free help if you're finding breastfeeding difficult; you can speak to a breastfeeding counsellor, who is a mum and who knows what you're going through

You don't have to be a member of the National Childbirth Trust (NCT) to call, but if you are interested in joining see the information in Chapter 9.

Expressing at work was difficult ... I was always sticky, and leaking. It was quite hard to guarantee that it [a nice room] would be there, so I often ended up expressing in the toilets, which wasn't very nice.

FY1 doctor

Breastfeeding advice that you won't find in a physiology textbook

Signs the baby is feeding well

- The baby is happy and seems relaxed, tucked in closely to your chest
- Her chin should be pressed into your breast, head back, and chin forward
- Her mouth should be wide open, with her bottom lip turned out
- There should be more breast in the baby's mouth below the nipple than above
- You should be able to see her face and jaw muscles working
- You can hear swallowing and gulping
- You can feel your 'let down' reflex; ranging from a warm, tingling feeling to slight discomfort, which goes away
- Do you feel happy and relaxed, are you enjoying the feed?

Warning signs

- Baby has 'pinched' lips
- Her cheeks are sucked in
- There are clicking noises
- You can hear lip-smacking
- It is not normal to feel pain that continues throughout the feed; don't listen to people who tell you this is normal. Seek help sooner rather than later.

I breastfed for about six weeks, but I gave it up for him [my partner] because he was having trouble bottle feeding when I wasn't there.

FY1 doctor

Help if you have sore nipples

- Make sure the baby is latching on properly; ask someone to watch you feed, such as your health visitor, your mum, or another mum

- Try changing the position you feed your baby—try with the legs under your arm, head forward, or feed lying down
- Use a specially designed cream (Vaseline is OK but not good enough long term, and Lamisol is better—before and after every feed)
- Don't use soap on your breasts in the shower
- If you need to take your baby off the breast before they've finished feeding, remember to release the suction (gently hook your little finger into the corner of their mouth)
- See your Health Visitor or GP if you think it may be thrush (especially if you experience a stabbing, sharp pain on feeding).

I went hunting around for somewhere to express [before I was due to go back to work]. I refused to express in the toilets ... So I went to the baby ward. I asked the sister, who bit my head off; she said she wasn't there to provide a service for expressing bloody doctors, and could I get off her ward unless I had a patient to see! I was a senior registrar at that point, and I couldn't believe she was speaking to me like that ... With a lot of persuasion, occupational health let me use one of their rooms; they used to reluctantly find me an office, and I used to trot back to clinic and put it in the fridge with everybody else's milk, and say 'Right, if you touch that, you're dead.'

Consultant surgeon

I was doing a theatre list ... I would get to the point where I was exploding, I'd try and wait'til between cases, but sometimes I just couldn't, and once I said 'Look I really need to go,' and my boss said 'Oh go, you unspeakable woman, get out before you make a mess ... And don't leak into the wound!'

Consultant surgeon

You may decide not to offer your baby a bottle, and choose to wean them straight from the breast to a beaker with a lid. This may be because you are not planning to return to work until your baby is fully weaned. You may, however, still breastfeed them if they wake up at night for many months to come; a milk feed may be the only way of getting them to go back to sleep.

Be aware that if your job involves doing nights, or even just late shifts, your baby will be waking up and you won't be there. Unless your partner has amazing gynaecomastia and some complicated surgery, he will be stuck with a screaming baby who wants you and only you.

With this in mind, it may be worth introducing a bottle of expressed milk once breastfeeding is established, just occasionally, so that the baby learns that it is another way of getting milk. Babies love breastfeeding; remember this if anyone tells you that you could 'ruin' your breastfeeding by giving the occasional bottle. Trying to introduce a bottle once the baby is a few months old is less likely to be successful.

Some more comments from doctors who have continued to breastfeed once they returned to work:

We tried a child minder first, but [the baby] wouldn't settle. We tried for about a month, and I came back working just mornings, because she wouldn't eat or drink at the child minders ... Then my mother had her for a bit ... Then we had a nanny. I was still breastfeeding when I came back to work, and she wouldn't take a bottle or take a cup, and we went through the most amazing traumas before I came back to work ... She wouldn't take any other fluid ... I would never do that again. I think once you get one established, you need to get the other going too ... I would feed her before I went to work, then she would last until lunchtime ... Then I would feed her when I collected her.

Consultant physician

You can still do on calls and breastfeed, even if they won't take a bottle. Mine wouldn't take any other fluid, other than breastfeeding, and they used to go all day without drinking ... But they were eating all sorts, and I would breastfeed them as soon as I got in the car at the end of the day. They don't die if they don't have a drink for twelve hours, and if they were really desperate, they would have drunk. Once or twice, my husband had to bring the baby to me when I was on nights, so I could feed her during my shift. The only problem was for the mum—I'd be queuing up for the expressing machine!

ST paediatrics

My mother in law is a GP [in Australia,] and had her children in the seventies ... When her second child, my husband, was born, she used to take him into work and breastfeed mid consultation if needed! I'm not really sure if that would work nowadays.

ST anaesthetics

The fact that I had problems breastfeeding, it means I'm a lot better at dealing with mums who are having problems ... When I see a baby, and it's not feeding properly, I'm more understanding.

GP

I breastfed all [three] of them ... The first one had expressed milk, but for the second and third ones, I realised that expressing my milk wasn't that important, and that they could have [formula] milk when I wasn't there ... But I learned how to express very quickly—sitting on the toilet, with a pump, and four minutes later, I was out of there!

Consultant surgeon

I had to give up [breast] feeding on my third one at eight months, because I had my FRCS to do, and your brain's not quite concentrating when you're feeding... I didn't want to have to worry about it when I was doing such a major exam.

Consultant surgeon

She still wakes me up a couple of times during the night for a breastfeed ... And it's really hard, if you're stressed out, and she wakes me up at 4am and I have to get up at five ... But it's worth it, it's really worth it.

FY1 doctor

References

National Childbirth Trust (September 2004) *Bumps and Babies*, Vol. 1, No. 12. National Childbirth Trust, London.

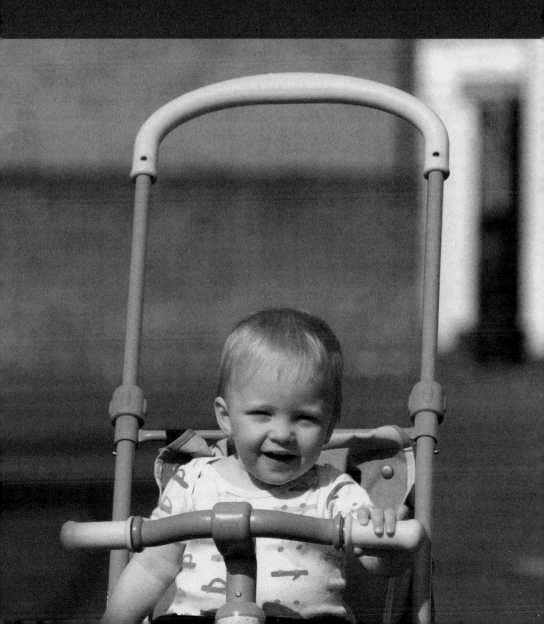

Chapter 14

Childcare

Oh god, I've left my children with the electrician, the plumber, the decorator ...

Consultant surgeon

Deciding on the type of childcare that will suit you and your family best can be a real source of stress. The conversation at 'baby massage' or at the playground will suddenly start to revolve around the fact that all the local nurseries have a waiting list of 10 years, or that all the Australian nannies are going back home because of changes to their visas. It's quite possible that, at this point, not only are you in denial about going back to work, but you're also in the dark about the difference between a nanny and a child minder.

To be honest, because I'd been at work before I was at medical school, it was much easier being a medical student with kids than being at work ... If something happens, if the child's sick, you just go ... Whereas at work, it just wasn't like that. You've got much more flexibility with your childcare as a student.

Medical student

If you work in hospital, or are a medical student, your Trust may have a Childcare Co-ordinator. What do they do?

- They are experts in childcare, dedicated to Trust employees
- They develop, implement, and evaluate childcare provision in order to meet the needs of employees
- They co-ordinate provision of nursery places, before and after school clubs, and holiday play schemes
- They promote the positive benefits of using child-minders
- They promote and encourage take-up of Child Tax Credit
- They promote Improved Working Lives (IWL)

In a nutshell, you should be able to call them through switchboard and discuss local options for childcare, and ask advice about covering odd shifts/school holidays etc

Once you know your childcare options, you can then start to plan your return to work. The best place to go for information is your local **Children's Information Service (CIS)**. Every local authority has a CIS, and it will tell you about the local childcare options available to you (they can usually give you information about the nursery at your local hospital too, even if it is only available for staff).

Home-based childcare: nannies and au pairs

Does the word nanny conjure up images of Mary Poppins, or of Bette Davis in the 1965 horror? Whatever your views are, if you want to work full-time in an acute medical speciality, or in surgery, and your partner works full-time too, a nanny or au pair is probably the best option.

What are they?

They are employed by you, to look after your child (or children) in your own home.

Positive points?

Great if you work unusual hours, as they often live with you, so can put your child to bed if you're working late, get them up in the morning, and cook their meals. Ideal if you have to work nights. Some will do other work around the house too, such as ironing and housework. They can be a cheaper option if you have more than one child, as you pay a set fee. Your child is able to be in his or her own home environment.

> We take Nanny on holiday with us ... Which is all very well, but I spend all my time trying to get her organized, so that she can organize the children. It's a rest to be back at work.
>
> *Consultant cardiologist*

Negative points?

They are not normally inspected by Ofsted. This is the Office for Standards in Education, the body which registers and inspects people who look after children aged under 8. Anyone can advertise themselves as a nanny, and they may not have any formal qualifications (such as nursery nurse training, or first aid). Unlike us, they don't have to be checked out by the Criminal Records Bureau, unless they are hired by an agency. You will have to pay not only their wages, but also their tax and National Insurance contributions. You are also responsible for holiday pay, sick pay, and you may decide to help with their mobile phone costs (for contacting you, not Australia), and it probably helps to add them to your car insurance.

> I worked four days a week in the City before I came to medical school ... My children were six and four, so they were both at school once I was a student; I think that took away some of the pressure. The difficulties I had were around getting them to school in the morning, and picking them up. [We had] a nanny who took them to school on a

Monday and picked them up, and did the same on a Friday. We had Wednesday afternoons off anyway, so that was ok ... [The other] mornings, I had to leave them with friends, or miss a lecture, just muddle through basically.

Medical student

What is an au pair?

Usually single and young, from abroad, they want to study English. They live with you, and help out with domestic chores for a maximum of 5 hours a day. They have 2 days off a week, and an allowance of about £50 a week, plus meals and a room that is their own. They have no training or registration, so you might feel nervous leaving them with your young baby, but they could be perfect for after school care.

[My ex-partner] moved away, and I thought 'Oh god, how am I going to do this,' so I've succumbed to an au pair ... She gets £70 a week, and for that she does two nights babysitting a week, the occasional weekend, and when I come home, my kids have been fed, my dinner's on the table, the house is clean and the ironing's been done!

Consultant physician, single mother

Important questions to ask at interview

- If they will be living in, ask about friends or boyfriends who may want to stay over, smoking, use of your internet and telephone, and make it clear where you stand from the start.
- If living out, do they live nearby? Do you have to pay for taxis to and from work, especially if you are working late or early shifts?
- Will they stay overnight when you are on nights?
- Will they babysit in the evenings?
- What would they do in a typical day? Where would they take your baby/child, what activities would they do?
- Ask about experience, training, first aid qualifications.
- Ask them why they want to do the job.

My husband is a Reg in A&E, so we have an au pair who lives in and puts the kids to bed. If I'm working late, I often don't make it home before they go to bed. She can cook their dinner, make sure everything's ok for them.

ST general practice

Agencies

The safest and easiest way of choosing a nanny or au pair is with an agency; use one that has a good reputation (ask around at work and where you live) and always check references. Any childcarer listed with them should have had a Criminal Records Bureau check, and may hold a basic first aid qualification; check with the agency. Talk to at least two previous employers, to get some idea of what other people think.

You can access agencies online (use a search engine to find sites). Refer to the 'Need a Nanny' guide on the Surestart website; http://www.surestart.gov.uk/about-surestart/.

It is essential to draw up a legally binding contract. It may also help to issue them with an unofficial 'parents contract', stating your views on diet, exercise, plus routines and bedtimes. You need to agree on discipline. Make sure they know how much TV your kids are allowed to watch, and how long they are allowed to spend playing computer games. If they are going to take your children out and about, make it clear how much they can spend on a typical day (the Sanctuary Spa is not essential for 5 year olds).

> I've always paid for a nanny. My husband works in a bank, so his hours are actually worse than mine! My older sister is a lawyer, and she's gone through a variety of childcare options, but I couldn't face putting them in to nursery and them always being the first ones there, and the last ones out; the 'Doctors Children!' I couldn't bear trying to put them in the car in their pyjamas at seven o clock in the morning, racing around trying to get myself ready.
>
> *Consultant surgeon*

> I think [having a nanny] is the only option for most doctors... They try other things out for the first child, get very stressed, but eventually they all come round.
>
> *Consultant surgeon*

> We have a nanny all year, she doesn't live in, she lives out, so school holidays are sorted ... And because she lives out, it means that when I'm not there, she is, but when I'm there, she isn't ... Which is perfect!
>
> *Consultant colo-rectal surgeon*

Average costs of a nanny

In the UK, costs vary locally, but the average rate is anything from £6.50 upwards per hour, and depending on whether you want someone who is going to teach your child Cantonese and yoga at the same time, the sky's the limit. A full-time place may vary from £250 (live-in, rural area) to £400 per week and more (live-out, central London,) and you will also have to pay tax and National Insurance on top of that amount.

For help with the financial aspects of employing a nanny, contact Nannytax, (http://www.nannytax.co.uk) a payroll support service for employers of nannies.

They provide unlimited support and advice on all pay- and employment-related issues and also offer free and comprehensive employment law support.

Average cost of an au pair

They are provided with a weekly allowance (about £50) and you need to provide them with their own room, and meals.

Before employing someone as a nanny or au pair, contact the HM Revenue and Customs' employers' helpline on 0845 6070 143.

The childcare element of the working tax credit should be applicable; see Chapter 19 'Money matters.'

Child-minders

If you usually only need childcare during the day, but need more flexibility than most nurseries can offer, a child-minder may be the perfect option. Some will be available for an occasional weekend or overnight, and your child will spend time in a normal family environment, often with the child-minder's own children.

> I went back part time three days a week to finish my modules, and I had a child-minder for the days I was at the hospital … I was lucky because [my husband], he had a job just down the road, where he didn't have to start until nine, so he could wait in for the child minder; she came to our house. But now, we have to get up at 5.30am, every morning, to get us all ready to leave before 7am, so we can drop her off at the child minder's … He has to be at work at eight now, same as me, and I have to travel a long way there.
>
> *FY1 doctor*

What are they?

A child-minder works in their own home, and will usually have other children, including their own, to look after. They can look after up to six children under the age of 8, but only three of them can be under 5.

Positive points?

Your child is cared for in a family environment, with children of different ages. Siblings of different ages can be looked after together. Child-minders can usually be more flexible than a nursery, and some do overnight stays or weekends. All adults (over 16's) living in the house will be police checked. Your child will be looked after by the same person, often for many years. All child-minders have to do a basic training course, which includes first aid. All child-minders are registered and inspected by Ofsted.

Negative points?

You could be in trouble if your child-minder is ill; however, most child-minding networks have something in place to ensure that if your child-minder is sick, another child-minder in the network may be able to help out. If there is a mix of young babies and older children, the babies have to go out on the school run. If your baby has a very strict routine, it may be difficult, as they have to fit in with the child-minder and his or her family. You still pay them if your child is ill and doesn't go, or if you have a day off with your child.

Visit more than one child-minder, to get a feel for things. Don't be embarrassed to tell each child-minder that you are visiting others. Be assertive, and say what you want for your child, and if it doesn't feel right, it probably isn't right.

Important questions to ask at interview

- How many other children will be with my child, and how old are they?
- Do you belong to a child-minding network?
- Where will my child sleep during the day?
- What kinds of meals and drinks do the children have?
- Are you happy to store frozen breast milk/use re-useable nappies (if applicable)?
- Do you have any pets?
- Do you, or does anyone else at home, smoke?
- Do you charge for sick days?
- What arrangements are in place in case you are unwell?
- What do you do on a typical day? Do they prefer 'routines' or are they happy for your child to sleep when they want to?
- Do you normally keep a communication diary for me to see, of what you did each day?

Settling in

All babies and children need a period of 'settling in' with a new care-giver. For nannies and au pairs, this could simply mean them spending time at home with the family. Most child-minders and nurseries will suggest a way of settling in, such as first staying with your child, then leaving the child for a short while but staying in the building, then leaving completely for an hour or so.

No one can prepare you for how you will feel. You may, like me, burst into tears at the bus stop, or you might relish your new found freedom and enjoy a few hours off!

However it is arranged, make sure you don't leave it until the last minute. You'll have enough to worry about when you re-start work, and settling in can take a week or two in some nurseries. In order for your child to feel safe and settled, they need you to be relaxed too.

A reasonable child-minder will not mind if you go back to visit them more than once. You may prefer to visit the first time without your child, just to get a feel for them and the place. Ask to see all the rooms in the house where your child will go, including the garden. It is also fine to ask for phone numbers of other parents, to call them and ask what they think of the child-minder. Child-minders usually provide all meals and snacks, but you usually provide milk and nappies.

Before you make any decisions, check:

- Their up-to-date registration documents, including police checks (and for other adults in the family), public liability insurance, car insurance, and first aid certificates.
- Who else will be in the house when your child is there.
- Make sure you agree on things such as TV, diet, and discipline procedures.
- How much holiday pay you have to pay them, and how much they take each year.

- National Child-minding Association (NCMA): 0800 169 4486
- ChildcareLink will provide you with a list of local child-minders in your area: 0800 096 0296

Average cost of a child-minder

Some charge by the hour, others by the day and half day. The average cost on the UK is about £2.80 per hour, but it can be as high as £7 an hour. The average cost of a full-time place for an under 2 is £132 a week.

There is a free education offer with child-minders (see later on in this chapter). The childcare element of the working tax credit is applicable—see Chapter 19 'Money matters.'

Day nurseries

If the thought of someone else living in your home fills you with horror, or if you don't have the space, a nursery can provide all day care in a safe, structured environment. Your child can spend the day making a mess and eating mud pies, and there may even be a nursery on site at the hospital.

He did one day in nursery, and my mother looked after him two days a week ... When I changed hospitals, he went to the hospital nursery ... They were very good, they were used to nurses and doctors, they were open seven'til seven, so when I was on call and did a mid-take ward round, he would be in for almost 11 hours... If we hadn't finished the ward round by seven, I took him out and took him to the emergency medical centre, where the nurses would entertain him ... There was one time we weren't going to finish on time, so my registrar kindly went and got him, then took him to the doctors mess, where everyone fed him chocolate biscuits, much to his delight!

Consultant physician

What are they?

They provide care and education for children from 6 weeks to 5 years, and may be operated by the council, your hospital, the community, or a private company.

He goes to nursery now. The nursery opens half seven in the morning, until six in the evening. I was offered a place in the hospital nursery, but that would have meant only me dropping him and taking him back. This is nearer the house; it means we can share it. We have to work our night shifts around each other... My husband is a paediatrician ... We try to swap [so we don't clash]. We have to take favours from our neighbour ... if we're running late, she can pick him up [from nursery].

ST medicine

Positive points?

Children can interact in large groups, cared for by trained staff. If the child's normal key worker is ill, someone else will look after them. Your child can attend full or part time, and they usually operate for 50 weeks of the year. Each child has their own key worker, who is their main carer. There will be lots of different activities and toys for them.

Negative points?

Siblings of different ages may be kept apart. The opening hours are strict, and they will not tolerate you being late, or trying to drop them off early. If your child doesn't have a routine, they may want them to sleep at certain times so they don't disturb the other children. You'll need a contingency plan for when your child is sick (and they'll pick everything up at nursery!) as unwell children can't attend nursery (ask each specific nursery for their definition of unwell—do they include loose stools in an otherwise well child?) You usually have set days, so it's difficult if you work on a rota where your days change. The children are usually in the same room all day, every day; not very stimulating. Timid children might find it a bit overwhelming at first.

Normal ratios of children to carers are three children per carer for under 2's, four children per carer for 2 year olds, and eight older children per carer.

Childcare Vouchers Scheme

- Some NHS Trusts allow their employees to take part of their salary in childcare vouchers. You essentially 'give up' part of your wages for the face value of the vouchers. The vouchers are non-taxable and are exempt from National Insurance contributions.

- Each £100 childcare voucher costs approximately £80 of your salary. Each family can take up to £6000 of vouchers per year.
- They cover all types of childcare (but all childcare providers who receive vouchers must be registered with Ofsted or an equivalent authority).
- Childcare vouchers can cover children up to the age of 16; for example for out of hours school clubs on school premises. They apply for foster children and legally adopted children too.
- The NHS Pensions Agency has confirmed that the value of the vouchers does not count as pensionable pay. As a result, you won't pay pension contributions on the value of the childcare vouchers you receive as part of your salary.
- The reduction in your salary will reduce the amount of your salary that is liable to National Insurance contributions; as a result, if you are expecting maternity leave, your Statutory Maternity Pay (SMP) may be reduced.
- The value of the childcare vouchers you receive will be ignored for calculation of Working Tax Credit or Child tax Credit (see Chapter 19) if you are 'sacrificing' part of your salary for the scheme. Discuss your circumstances with the Inland Revenue via their helpline (0845 300 3900).
- Contact your Trust's Childcare Co-ordinator for more information.

Important points to check at a nursery

- Do they provide emergency cover at short notice?
- What is their definition of an unwell child (i.e. when can't they come)?
- How many children does each carer look after?
- Can someone else (e.g. a named friend) collect your child if you're late?
- Is there a safe outdoor play area?
- Will a daily diary be kept?
- Ask to see a menu.
- What happens if you're late—are there penalties?
- Ask about trips out.
- What if my child doesn't have a routine?
- Ask to see where the children sleep.
- Will they use re-useable nappies and expressed breast milk?

Advantages of having a nursery/childminder near home

- Easier if you have an early start and you want your child to have breakfast once they get to nursery/the child-minder.
- You don't have to do the commute to work in the rush hour with a buggy or sling and a potentially miserable child.
- If public transport goes awry or your car gets stuck in traffic, it may drive you mad but it doesn't mean you have to cope with it and a child.
- Once you get your child, at the end of a long day, you're nearly home. You may both be tired and grumpy!
- If you are stuck at work or on your journey, a neighbour or friend may agree to act as an emergency contact and collect your child for you. (A nursery or childminder will usually only allow you or your partner to collect your child, unless you give written agreement for a named person, who will have a password, to collect them in exceptional circumstances.)

Advantages of having a nursery/childminder near work

- If your child is unwell you can get to them quickly.
- You are more likely to be able to pick your child up on time; some nurseries operate an extremely strict deadline for collection.
- You can spend more time with your child if you have a long journey to work.
- Your child may end up being with children of colleagues; this could be useful if there was an emergency and you absolutely couldn't get away on time.
- Colleagues may know the local childcare options well, and may be able to advise you on those who are prepared to be more flexible.

I used to have to belt back every single day... I was still with my partner, but he was working somewhere else ... Then he would say. 'Well you're part time, you can get away to get the kids,' and I thought well, yes, but you never have to rush away, I'm always breaking my neck to leave at ten to five.

Consultant physician

Nursery opened at half seven in the morning, and closed at six, so I was always clock-watching at the end of the day. At one point, when I moved jobs, she was in two separate nurseries on different days of the week.

Consultant physician

Some hospitals have a nursery on site; in contrast to other nurseries, they may open for up to 12 hours a day. If you're breastfeeding, you may be able to visit for feeds during the day (see Chapter 13). Fees are often based on what you earn, which is great if you're working part-time. The staff may be slightly more understanding about you being late to pick up, but still check if there are penalties. Some can provide emergency care.

National Day Nurseries Association (NDNA): 0870 774 4244

Before you make a final decision about a nursery, it may be helpful to go back and visit again, taking your child with you to see how they get on with the staff and the other children. Visit at a different time of day, and maybe try to speak with some of the other parents, to see what they think of the nursery.

Mums and mothers-in-law

Love them or loathe them, they could really save the day when it comes to childcare. Some parents are happy being at a distance, but for others it's the chance they've been waiting for and their reason for existing.

We've taught him [my 20 month-old son] to have a really long sleep in the middle of the day, for three or four hours, so he can stay up late and see me after work... My mother-in -law lives with us, she looks after him, because I work full-time. He goes to bed at about 9pm.

ST general practice

What are they?

The person who raised you (or your partner), and nagged you constantly about devoting too much time to your career instead of having children.

Positive points?

They might be free of charge, and they are madly in love with your child. They are genetically programmed to look after them. You don't have to flap around getting the child dressed and ready in the morning, and you know that your child will be delighted to spend time with her. If you are late from work you don't need to panic, as she can feed the child and put them to bed. If your baby is poorly you know you can still go to work. You can (hopefully) communicate freely with her, and tell her exactly what you want her to do, but ...

> My mother in law came to this country, to look after my children while I was working full time... But we didn't get on; it was a really awful time, in the end we had to send her back home... I said 'No-one's going to break up this family.'
>
> *ST geriatrics*

Negative points?

They might have their own ideas about raising your offspring, and may not listen to your instructions; unlike a childminder or nanny, you don't employ them, and you possibly don't pay them, so your ability to control what they do is limited. If you don't get on with them, it could all turn into a horrible mess. Some women feel that they 'take over.' They may have no idea about modern child rearing, or first aid, and they may stubbornly refuse to learn how to use their mobile phone, restricting your ability to stay in touch from work. If they end up moving in with you, it could cause marital discord. There is a chance that, unless she takes the child out and about, they won't get to socialize as much as if they were with a childminder or in a nursery. You may find that you struggle with feelings of gratitude for all her hard work, but envy her because she gets to spend all her time with the baby instead of you.

> My baby is in India, he lives with my mum, I get to see him in my holidays ... My mum stayed with me in England for the first six months, but then she had to go back there, and take him with her ... He's a year old now. But I can't go and see him in this time off; I've got to study for my exams.
>
> *ST paediatrics*

> We pay my mother-in-law to come over and look after our children ... We pay her the same as we would pay a nanny. She didn't want to take the money, but we insisted; I still need to feel like their mum, and we said that if she didn't want to keep the money, she could spend it on taking the children out, or she could put it in an account for the children. It's great, because I don't have to be clockwatching at the end of the day, if I'm stuck in resus in a trauma call, I'm not worrying about getting out on time... The worst thing about it is she ends up doing bits of housework, unlike a nanny would, and I find she's washed my underwear, which is a bit weird!
>
> *ST paediatric A&E*

Partners

My own father didn't know one end of a nappy from the other, but thank goodness, times have changed. It is now increasingly common for dads to stay at home full time, or to work part time, and spend more time bringing up their children.

What are they?

The other half of the zygote.

Positive points?

Probably too many to mention; apart from being the child's father, if you can afford it then it can be wonderful for the whole family.

Negative points?

They don't usually clean the kitchen as well as au pairs (I know, that's controversial). You may find your feelings of guilt, and jealousy, actually increase, if you feel you are 'missing out.' The shift in power in the relationship can cause stormy waters, especially if your partner gave up a very prestigious job in order to stay at home.

> I found it awfully difficult to leave work on time to get to the childminder's; especially when you had an interesting patient to follow up ... In the end, we decided that my husband would give up his job. It was a huge relief to me.
>
> *Consultant radiologist*

Nursery schools and classes

One day you're tearing your hair out over how and when to go back to work and leave your tiny baby, then before you know it your child is ready to go to nursery school. Some take children from 2, whereas others are for 3–5 year olds. They provide early education, and may be run by the state, a private organization, or the voluntary sector.

What are they?

They provide learning and development activities from 9 a.m. to 3.30 p.m. in term time, and some provide extended hours for working parents.

Positive points?

They are regularly inspected by Ofsted, and if you're in the catchment area for a state nursery, the care may be free, but only for about 2 hours a day (a part-time place). All classes are run by qualified teachers. There is continuity of care, and your child will get to meet other local children.

Negative points?

Despite being free for a couple of hours, it may be no good if you are working long hours. You may feel that it's too much structure, at too early an age.

Make sure you try and visit the nursery school during a teaching session, in order to see the children interacting with the staff. Always go back for a second visit, and take your child along.

> The free nursery place was only for two hours a day... That was no good ... So my kids went to a private nursery

Consultant physician

Questions to ask

- Ask about staff turnover.
- Are there arrangements for your child to sleep if they need to?
- How do I go about settling my child in?
- What is a typical day?
- Is there an outside play area?
- Are there additional costs, such as meals and trips?
- Do you keep a daily record of each child?

Babysitters

There may be occasions when you are stuck trying to cover an evening shift, or to bridge a gap between you leaving for work in the evening, and your partner coming home. It may help to find a good, local babysitter, that you can call on if you need to, if your usual childcare is only in the daytime. It hurts, because it's expensive. They may be earning more than you, while lounging on your sofa with their boyfriend, but in times of need, it may be your only choice.

If friends and neighbours offer to help out, you can feel incredibly guilty when you do have to call on them. But remember that most mums will, at some point, have to leave their child with the neighbour's mum, or the builder, while they race off to a job interview or to teach students. A big box of chocolates or a bunch of flowers usually does the trick, and they usually, genuinely, don't mind.

Free part-time early education for 3–4 year olds

From April 2006, all 3 and 4 year olds have been entitled to a free part-time early education place. It counts for five sessions a week, of 2 and a half hours duration, for 38 weeks a year.

The places are available in school nursery classes, state or private nursery schools, day nurseries, playgroups and pre-schools, and with accredited child-minders who are part of a network. It is not available to help with the cost of a nanny or au pair.

For more information, contact your local Children's Information Service (CIS) via ChildcareLink on 0800 096 0296.

References

Department for Education and Skills (2006) *Looking for Childcare? A Surestart guide to help you make the right choices*. DfES Publications, Nottingham. www.surestart.gov.uk/aboutsurestart/parents/lookingforchildcare

Chapter 15

Being back at work

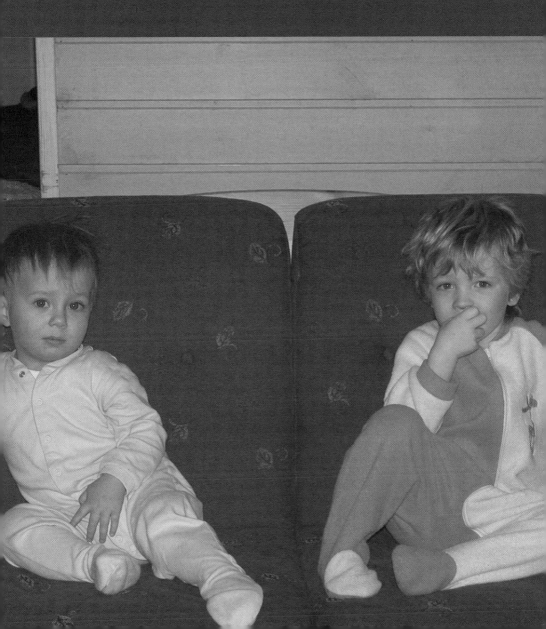

The first day I went back [to work after having my baby] I kept ringing home, because I felt that I should, rather than because I felt I needed to, because I was a bit shocked at how easily I had just slotted back into work ... And you just get on with work, and you're in a different mould to being 'mum.'

GP

Finding your GMC certificate could take some time (but once resurrected may or may not be ripped/scribbled on/peed on by your toddler), and occupational health may need some reassurance that you still have a BCG scar, even after all these months off, but before you know it you'll be facing your first day back at work. If you're going back to your old job, in the same hospital or practice as before, you can relax in the knowledge that most of the day will be taken up showing everyone pictures of the baby. If you're changing jobs though, the day can be quite daunting; not only do you have to meet new colleagues, new patients, and maybe even get your head around a new speciality, but you may feel that your brain is still in the labour ward.

She was only five weeks old when I went to my first lecture, because I was doing a taught course, and I had to do two lectures a week ... I stood on the station platform crying ... But then I thought, well, the reason for my life is her, but the reason for her life wasn't me ... And so we'd better get used to being apart pretty quickly ... And then I was fine! I decided I could either cry for the afternoon, or have a hot cup of coffee ... I had a coffee, and some cake, and had a thoroughly enjoyable lecture!

Consultant colo-rectal surgeon

Advice that might help you get to work on time

- Decide what you and your child are going to wear the night before, and leave it out.
- Get your handbag ready the night before; if you need to take lunch with you, make it the night before.
- If your child goes to a nursery/childminder, pack their bag the night before (you'll usually need spare clothes, nappies, milk, and sometimes their lunch too).
- Don't get too stressed if your child won't eat breakfast in the morning; they won't starve to death.
- If your young baby enjoys possetting large volumes of milk, hang your work clothes up by the front door. Do all your organizing in scruffy clothes, and

get changed just as you are about to leave (even once the baby is strapped into the buggy).

- Plan to leave the house 10 minutes before you actually have to leave the house.

- If your child does a poo/gets a nosebleed/has a tantrum just as you're opening the front door, remember that you'll probably still get there on time; if it's looking unlikely, call work and explain. The world will not stop turning.

- The above advice is evidence-based, gold standard. It is impossible to stick to, and most of us end up leaving the house with a bawling child covered in weetabix, wearing yesterday's clothes. Good luck.

Even the most confident woman can feel nervous about being back at work. If you had a traumatic delivery, you might even find it difficult being back in a hospital, or dealing with pregnant patients in the surgery. You may not have opened a copy of the BMJ since you went on leave, and suddenly you're expected to slot back into place with all your clinical skills and knowledge intact.

> The first few days were the hardest, because I was doing a really quiet firm … it made me want to be at home all the time, it seemed a waste to be there when we weren't doing anything. My medicine job is really busy, but it's better in a way—although I'm away longer, I'm busy, so it's not so hard being away.
>
> *FY1 Medicine*

> I was absolutely terrified of there being a trauma call, I just felt like I shouldn't be there … Everyone else seemed so confident, just getting on with it, and I felt like I didn't know anything.
>
> *FY2 medicine*

Try to remember that you are not the first woman to have gone on maternity leave. If you feel lacking in knowledge, remember that you have acquired a great deal of knowledge in the fields of obs and gynae, and paediatrics. Your confidence will come back with time, and as soon as you've recovered from the shock of someone calling you 'doctor', you'll be back into the swing of things.

Having trouble with your confidence on returning to work?

- Remember that you are not the first doctor to return after a long period of leave; doctors of both sexes go on extended sick leave, take sabbaticals, and change specialities.

- Although it might sound like madness, working towards an exam may actually increase your confidence.
- Go on a course.
- Talk to other female doctors who have done the same thing.
- Keep you head up, and remember that you are a qualified doctor; you really did pass your exams!

Medicine is stressful enough, and I don't think you need your colleagues frowning on you when you are pregnant, or frowning on you when something happens with your childcare, and yet they do ... Some of them are not very understanding ... They don't understand the pressure it is trying to do your job well and also have a family.

Consultant physician

How do I leave work on time?

Medicine is not a 9–5 job, and there will never be enough doctors on the ward to do all the work in the time available. Your surgery finishes when the last person leaves, and emergencies need to be dealt with there and then. Before you had children, you probably just stayed, and the hardest thing in the world is trying to get away on time to collect your baby from nursery.

Medicine is a job you can't put down at five o clock, but for colleagues, they need to recognize that, if a mother has to go and pick up a child, she just has to go ... Shift work, with the European Working Time Directive, may actually be beneficial to mothers who want to work in a hospital speciality ... If they know someone is coming in to take over, it might make a real difference ... If there were clearer boundaries [as to what time you started and finished work], it might be more manageable.

ST2 medicine

My registrar, she was organized down to a tee, but if she didn't leave at five, it all fell apart.

ST1 medicine

I'm supposed to work three and a half days a week, but by leaving on time on a Monday in order to pick him up from nursery, I never get away on time Friday lunchtime, so I usually miss my half day.

GP

Trying to leave work on time to collect your children

• Remember that you're leaving in order to collect your children, not go to the pub; most reasonable people don't mind.

• It might help to remind people, at the start of the day, that you need to get away on time and why, rather than panic at 5 p.m.

• As a hospital doctor, there should be someone to hand over to; remember that when you're on call, people hand things over to you, that's the point! Organize your hand over early and don't try and bleep them 1 minute before you need to leave.

• If you have to sit in a meeting that is supposed to finish at 5, say at the beginning that you need to leave on time and why.

• Remember that before you had children, you didn't understand why this was all so important; people without children naturally find it hard to understand the difference between leaving at 5.15 p.m. and leaving at 5.45 p.m.

I can never get out on time, I can never guarantee it. I hate getting home and he's gone to bed, and I haven't seen him all day. That's the hardest bit.

GP

Surviving your new life as a doctor and a mum can be difficult at times. The worst thing, apart from when they are ill, is when your child wakes you up every night. You can spend your days feeling slightly 'jet lagged,' and after a while the chronic effects of sleep deprivation can make you feel terrible. Teaching your baby that night time is for sleeping, not for drinking milk or creeping into bed with you, is difficult, but worth it.

Sleep problems (the baby, not you)

I'm not Gina Ford, and I never read any of her baby books. I believe that mums know what is best for them and their babies, and shouldn't feel guilty if they think they're not doing the 'right' thing. If you think the following isn't right for you, then don't do it.

Before I was pregnant, I used to say that I'd never leave a baby to cry. 'Sleep training,' or 'controlled crying' seemed the worst thing in the world you could do. Once you've had a child though, you realize that if you are constantly woken up all night, for months on end, you can feel like you're going to die. If you're trying to cope with work at the same time, it can really kill you.

Once your baby is about 5 or 6 months old, if you want to teach them how to go to sleep, and how to sleep through the night, you could try 'controlled crying.' I think I cried more than the baby when I did it, and don't let anyone tell you it's easy, but it was the best thing I ever did; suddenly, I had evenings again, and could usually get a decent night's sleep.

If you're going to do it, make sure you have a week or so when nothing much is planned in the evenings; it could really ruin a dinner party. Try and have someone around to support you.

How to do it (there are other ways; ask your health visitor if you need advice or support):

1. Remember that your baby loves you.

2. Tell your neighbours what you are doing.

3. Remember that babies do not explode, even if they cry for a long time.

4. Put your baby to bed after a bit of a 'routine' (bath, story, milk).

5. Kiss them goodnight, and walk out of the room.

6. They will cry. Leave them for 5 minutes.

7. Go back in, reassure them with confidence, and walk out again.

8. Leave them for 10 minutes

9. Repeat, increasing the amount of time between going in by 5 minutes.

10. In between, don't sit on the top stair bawling and listening to them cry. Go into a room as far away as possible, put on some loud music, watch the TV, whatever works.

Some babies will cry for a couple of hours on the first night. It is horrendous, and you may feel terrible, but you must stick to it or it won't work. It isn't natural for you to leave a crying baby, and it is designed to make you feel awful! The next night, they probably won't cry as long. If you are consistent, this method usually only takes a few nights to work. You might then be able to put your baby down, walk out, and find that they go straight to sleep. The older the baby is, the more stamina they have, and the harder they pull at your heart strings.

I'm quite tired, really tired, but I just love it. I love her so much. I wouldn't change a thing.

FY1 doctor

Taking exams

Revision will take on a whole new meaning once you've got children, but that doesn't mean it's impossible. You need to be good at time management and be very focused;

gone are the days when you could sit at the dining room table, staring into space, wondering what to wear when you go out later. If you can't afford any extra child care, then you need to structure your work around when the baby sleeps. This might be difficult if your baby is small and only sleeping on you during feeds in the daytime, or waking up lots in the evening for feeds. Once they're bigger, you'll struggle if they'll only have a daytime sleep in the pram (which is being pushed around the park at 30 miles an hour). My baby could sense when the pram had stopped, and I spent a long time wondering how there were mothers who could sit and drink coffee, or read a paper, while their baby slept soundly in a stationary pram. The key is to try and get the baby to sleep in their bed in the daytime, or at least somewhere that's not on top of you, so you can actually get some work done. The sleep training, as described above, was the key to me having time in the evenings. My life was transformed once my baby went to bed at seven o'clock and (usually) stayed there! If doing work at home is non-starter, then you'll just have to try and do what you can while you're at work. Take books in for quiet days, and grab every opportunity you can for teaching.

> It was hard with exams and stuff [when both my partner and I were taking them] because my partner would go to all the teaching and everything but I was missing out big style because I had to go and get the baby ... it didn't seem right.
>
> *Consultant physician*

On the day of an exam, it's nice to have extra help with your children, but you might not be able to arrange it. If you can, ask a kind relative or friend to help you in the morning, so you can get yourself ready and leave the house without rice crispies in your hair or diprobase on your suit. Charging down to nursery can leave you feeling frazzled on any day, but if you've got to get yourself to somewhere miles away in order to sit an exam, it can be a nightmare. (See Chapter 6, 'Pregnancy as an undergraduate', for further advice.)

There are certain specialities that take on a whole new meaning once you're a mum. If you had a difficult birth, working on labour ward may be very stressful at first. If your baby was in special care, going on to SCBU may make you want to cry. And working in paediatrics is definitely different if you have a family of your own. My first trauma call, when I was working in paediatric A&E, was to a toddler who was the same age as my own. He'd been brought in by the helicopter after a huge television had fallen on his head. I found myself trying not to cry for the first hour or so, and found it impossible to dissociate myself from the scene in front of me. I then had to spend the following weekend at my parents' house, with my child rushing up to the enormous, precariously balance television (which she'd never taken much notice of before), trying to grab hold of it. I was a nervous wreck after a few days.

> My children were quite small when I was working in paeds A&E ... It was really quite distressing; I struggled a bit whenever I saw a really sick child.
>
> *GP*

I do a lot of paeds, the eczema clinic, and I used to say ridiculous things to parents [before I had children], like 'You must stop them scratching!' Now, those clinics are transformed for me, I've got insight, and the parents trust me more ... I'm definitely a better doctor ... But every time I have to go to paediatric intensive care, to biopsy a child, I get very upset; I can't get my head around it really.

Consultant dermatologist

Advice if you are a single mum/if your partner works away for periods of time/if your partner is a doctor and your night shifts clash

If you have a nanny or an au pair who lives with you, then being on your own is easier to manage. If you need to do nights, or late shifts, or an unexpected weekend session, you should be able to organize the childcare.

If your children only have day care, then you may need a contingency plan to cover your shifts, or your late surgeries.

- Do you know other mums who have a live in nanny or au pair? Would they come to some financial agreement and allow your child to sleep over night for the odd week when you have to work nights?
- If you are working nights, remember that you'll need some child care during the day in order to let you get some rest.
- Could your mum, sister, or a good friend stay at your home the nights you're away? Could your child stay overnight with a good neighbour?

[My ex partner] lived down the road, so he would have them when I was on call, else I would have struggled with the on calls. They were a lot heavier in those days, if I'd been a full time reg ... So I did flexible training ... Seven sessions ... When they changed to shift patterns, it was a bit hard. I used to say 'Let me do every Wednesday,' then whoever was on could have the night off, everyone was fine with it, because I was totally supernumerary. [Medical] staffing were fine, so I did the right amounts, but I picked my days, everybody was happy with that ... I could choose nights that my ex-partner was off.

Consultant physician, single mother

I do four days a week, but the same on call as my colleagues, one in four. Weekends, Saturday and Sunday morning, it means coming in.

We usually box and cox it [my husband and I], because he's a surgeon, he looks after her [when I go in to work]. There has been the odd Saturday morning when she's had to come in to work with me, when my husband's been called in acutely, unexpectedly, something really urgent.

Consultant physician

Everybody talks about morning sickness; when I was pregnant, I was constantly asked whether I was being sick, even though I felt fine. Yet nobody warned me about 'toddler sickness'. I must have spent weeks with my head in a bucket by now. Sometimes it can feel that your child is constantly unwell, especially in the first few years of life; just as they recover from each new bug, and have lots of energy again, you come down with it. There will be days when you just can't juggle it, but if your colleagues have children of their own, they should understand what you're going through.

Parental leave

- Parental leave is unpaid leave of 13 weeks per parent, per child, which can be taken before the child's fifth birthday.
- If you are an adoptive parent, you can take it either within 5 years of placement for adoption, or before the child turns 18, whichever is earlier.
- If your child is on Disability Living Allowance, the leave is 18 weeks, to be taken before the child is 18.
- A part-time worker's entitlement is pro-rata.

My daughter got rotavirus within a week of me going back to work …

Consultant physician

When you don't have a Registrar (which is six months of the year for us in this job), or when you have a clinic, or when no one will do your work, or you've got a big family case conference lined up, or when you've got to do an interview, it's stressful … She was ill when I was supposed to be doing registrar interviews … I just had to ring the chairman of panel and say 'Look, I really can't leave her,' she had a temperature and was very unwell, I just couldn't leave her. She was small then, now I would have had to give her some calpol and get her out the door.

Consultant geriatrician

[If the baby is ill], if I've got a clinic fully booked, I guess it's like anything really … You just botch it … But when they're little, they just get everything, and I used to feel so, so guilty; the amount of times I'd have to ring up, and just say sorry, he's ill. They either have to cancel your clinic, or whoever else is in tries to 'mop up' your patients… It happens all the time in general practice. It doesn't faze me anymore.

GP

The hard work will all be worth it; one day you'll look back on what you've achieved, as a doctor and a mum, and be amazed at how you coped. There might be days when you think it's not worth it, you're totally exhausted, and you don't know whether you're doing the right thing. You're sick of clockwatching, trying to leave on time, and trying to maintain a happy home life and a relationship with your partner. Remember that you are, without a doubt, a superwoman. You've worked hard to be where you are, and you deserve to be there.

Some final words on being back at work

It's very levelling, to come home after a serious day at work, to be greeted by your toddler shouting 'mummy will you come and wipe my bottom?!

Consultant dermatologist

I've never been anywhere since she was born [to meetings or conferences] … other than in [this city] … even now I can't go away overnight, she won't leave me. I think because she was so unhappy at the child minders at the beginning, she's very clingy, even now.

Consultant physician

Going back full time wasn't too bad, as it was the shift system; I knew it was only for four weeks, so I just gritted my teeth and did it … To work full time only gave me the extra money to pay for the childcare; if I had him in nursery full time; so working as a flexible trainee worked well, as my family were able to help out.

Consultant physician

Although my colleagues are all men, they all have wives, and they have children, so their wives are in a similar position to me.

Consultant physician

It was a really grim time, actually … There wasn't quite enough of me to go around with my first child, but then my second came along, and the time I was at work, I wanted to be at home, and the time I was at home, I felt like I should be at work ... You've got this joint commitment, to your family and your patients, and sometimes the family had to come first, but sometimes my patients had to come first ... And I was deeply unhappy. So when my second child was about four months old, I went part time ... I did a job share [at registrar level], and that was just fantastic.

Consultant surgeon

When it came to applying for a consultant post, I just thought 'oh god, look at me, single mum, part timer, no research since my BSc, wow, I'm looking really good on paper here' ... But I've done it!

Consultant renal physician

People look at you differently when you have children ... One of my colleagues shocked me, when I came back from maternity leave, by saying 'Oh, I thought you were more ambitious than that ...' And I thought well, I think I've done alright actually, I'm a consultant in a teaching hospital ... And I've got the best of both worlds; I've also got a beautiful daughter.

Consultant physician

My baby was a beautiful sleeper, she'd just conk out ... I remember doing a locum at a small peripheral hospital, where I knew I had a four hour shift to cover without childcare. I decided to take her in to the reporting room with me, fast asleep in her basket, and I reported radiographs in the dark while she slept! I think my colleagues thought it was a bit strange, especially the supervisor, who was very old fashioned ... Remember that these were the days when he'd greet you, and help you on with your white coat, and bring you a tray of tea and biscuits on an embroidered cloth!

Consultant radiologist

References

British Medical Association (April 2007) *Maternity Leave (for NHS medical staff)*. Membership guidance note—NHS employment. British Medical Association, London.

Chapter 16

Working fathers

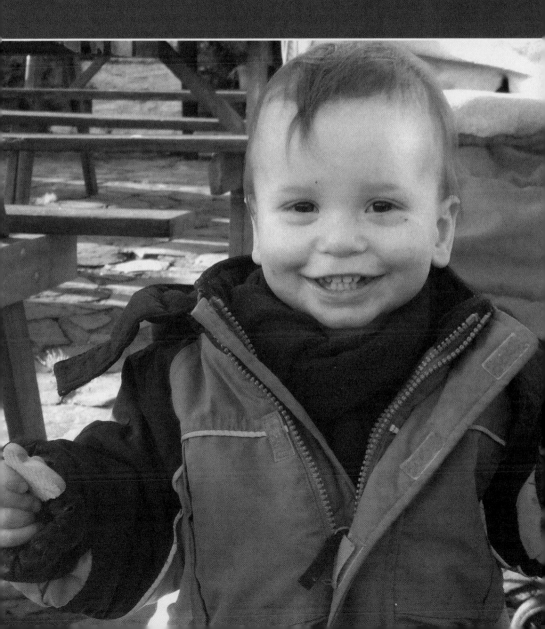

I mean, all this paternity leave rubbish ... When my wife had our son, it was on a Friday, and I was on call from Friday morning until Monday evening ... Everyone at work knew I had just had a baby. But I didn't see him until he was four days old. That's just the way it was.

Consultant surgeon

Since 2003, any man who has responsibility for the upbringing of a baby (defined as the biological father, or the mother's husband or partner if they are not the father) has been entitled to paternity leave. Same sex partners are also included. The law does not take into account the number of hours you work, but you must have worked for the same employer for 26 weeks ending with the 15th week before the baby is due, and from the 15th week before a baby is due, up to the time of the birth. The law states that you can take the time off to 'support the mother or care for the new baby,' so no sloping off to the pub or playing golf.

- Either 1 week, or 2 consecutive weeks, can be taken. You are not allowed to take the odd day off here and there.
- Twins (or more) do not mean that you get more time off.
- Your leave can start on the day the baby is born, or at a later day.
- You should have notified your employer (through HR in hospital, as well as telling your consultant if you are junior; in general practice you need to ensure the partners are all aware). This needs to be done by the end of the 15th week before the baby is due but exceptions can be made if you inform them at a later date.

In retrospect, I would have done things differently. I was starting my first consultant post, I was moving house, and I was having my first baby. I found it all extremely difficult, and got a bit frayed around the edges! When you're a new consultant, you want to be really enthusiastic, and positive, and I just kept getting ill all the time ... I took a week or so of paternity leave, right at the beginning, when he was about a week old ... But that wasn't the right time to take it. They're just sleeping all the time, or feeding... And there are all these other people around too, parents and friends, I felt a bit useless really ... And lots of people ringing up. I should have taken it once he was a few months old, when you're completely exhausted and sleep deprived ... Or when you partner goes back to work, that would be a good time to take it.

Consultant, infectious diseases and medical microbiology

Statutory Paternity Pay

If you are eligible for paternity leave, then you may also be eligible for paternity pay. It is paid at the same rate as statutory maternity pay, which at the time of writing is

£112.75 per week, or 90% of your average weekly earnings if this is a lesser amount. Rather than going through pregnancy and labour, however, you simply need to make sure that you:

1. Tell your employer that you want Statutory Paternity Pay 28 days beforehand, in writing (write to HR, and write to your consultant, and in general practice write to the other partners).
2. State the Estimated Date of Delivery of the baby, in terms of the week it is due, whether you want to take 1 or 2 weeks leave, and when you want to start your leave.
3. Make a signed declaration that you are taking the leave to care for the mother or the baby or both, that you expect to have responsibility for the upbringing of the child, and that you are either the biological father of the child, or are the mother's husband or partner. In other words, I promise I'm not going to come back from this leave with a ski-goggles suntan.

Once you've had your paternity leave, you'll be back at work and wondering where the time went. I think that as women we often forget the implications of being a doctor and being a new dad; having to start early and finish late, and going for days without seeing your child if you're on late shifts. People often ask how the mother is in the early days, whereas you might be struggling to come to terms with the fact that you're a dad. If your selective deafness allows you to sleep next to a screaming baby in a Moses basket, then at least you'll get a good night's rest. If, however, you're woken up every time the baby wakes up, then you'll probably need a caffeine infusion to keep you going at work the next day.

> I always do his bottle when he wakes up in the night... Otherwise I would never get to see him; I'm at work all day long, and never get to spend any quality time with him.
>
> *ST medicine*

> Yes, I remember all the screaming in the evenings ... I think it was around that time that I decided to start doing evening out-patient clinics.
>
> *Consultant orthopaedic surgeon*

If you're working in hospital medicine, and you're working nights, it can be hard to get rest during the day, even with older children. Just as you're nodding off, your baby may decide he doesn't actually enjoy having his nappy changed, and screams blue murder in the room next door. If the weather's bad, then your partner or nanny might not be too pleased about spending the day in the playground in the pouring rain.

> It's difficult trying to sleep in the daytime, when I've been on nights ... They try and make themselves scarce [my partner and the baby] but it's not easy, trying to sleep, when they're downstairs.
>
> *ST geriatrics*

Women aren't the only ones to discover that being a parent makes you a different doctor. Whereas previously, you might have been annoyed by the parents of children fussing and fretting about 'minor' problems, bringing their children to A&E with microscopic scalp lacerations. They might still annoy you, but now you can probably see why the parents are so anxious. 'I haven't slept for three nights because of the baby' takes on a whole new meaning, and at last you can finally undo those weird babygros and put a nappy back on properly.

> My husband [a general and colo-rectal surgeon] always sees the kids first on the ward round now; he understands how important it is since we've had children.
>
> *ST paediatrics*

If you still want to roll your eyes when parents turn up at emergency appointments with a child whose only problems are too much snot and too much energy, then maybe you'll find that you're more understanding of your colleagues, when they have to leave a ward round because nursery's sending their child home, or when they catch every virus under the sun from their very own 'biological germ bank.'

> When I think back to when I was a reg [before I had children], I was so insensitive to my colleagues who had kids... I remember, a couple was having problems with childcare, their au pair or something, and I remember just thinking 'Oh come on, it can't be that hard to sort out...' I'm much more understanding now, when my juniors are struggling.
>
> *Consultant, infectious diseases and medical microbiology*

> He always looks so smug because he's in early every day, and I'm always late... Just wait, when his baby's born, he won't make it in on time, ever.
>
> *ST urology*

Some dads decide to work part time, and unlike dads of my father's generation (who might have been labelled as a hippy, or unemployable) the man of the 'noughties' can stay at home without too many comments from the neighbours. They may be seen as big kids who want to play computer games all day, but making the decision to stay at home, and perhaps leave a lucrative career, can't be easy. While it's generally accepted that women may want to have time out from a career, or work part time, men may find it harder to get back into work at a later stage, or may be looked down on if they come from a profession that is highly competitive and male dominated.

> My husband had given up work, and I was a full time doctor. We'd go to dinner parties, and people would say to my husband 'So what do

you do?' and would never ask me ... Then he would explain our situation, and people would say 'Oh, how interesting!'

Consultant radiologist

Want to train flexibly?

A survey by the Conference of Postgraduate Medical Deans in 2006 revealed that only 3.9% were men. Just 4% of flexible trainees in the SpR grade were male, the figure rose to 5% at SHO grade, and 6% in the Foundation Years (Trueland, 2006).

See Chapter 12 for more information on part-time working.

References

Trueland J (2006) In a twist over flexible training. *BMA News*, **23 September**.

Chapter 17

'Planning' further pregnancies

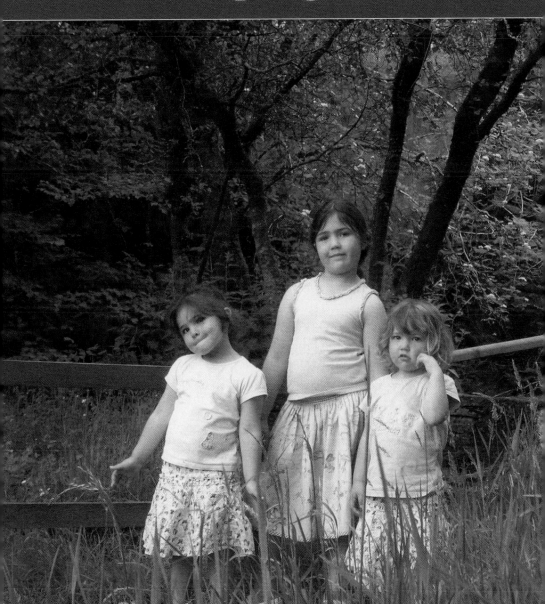

> I've been limited to four kids by my husband … there's no way he'd let me have any more!
>
> *ST general practice*

As I discussed at the start of the book, 'planning' does imply that one has a certain degree of control over a situation. Trying not to get pregnant is one thing, but trying to time a second pregnancy so that it fits into your career, your partner's career, and your existing family, is quite another. You'll have plenty of things to take into account, such as how long you want the gap between your children to be, how completely exhausted you feel, and how enthusiastic you both are about 'doing it all over again.' If you're nearing the end of your training, you may want to hold off for a little while until you're a GP or consultant; if you're a medical student, you might feel that you need to get your Finals over with before you embark on another pregnancy.

> There's a consultant, he's notorious for saying '… Oh for god's sake, please tell me that you're not going to get pregnant now you've gone and got your number … He said to my friend, who had just come back to work after having her first baby, 'I hope you're going to wait for several years before you have another baby, don't have any more time off yet.'
>
> *ST medicine*

Other women may want to have their children close together, at the start of their training, so that once they attain the higher ground of consultant or GP, they can concentrate on their career rather than having to take time out. Being part time in a very junior grade can be a bit soul destroying at times, as you see all your peers race ahead. As a part-time doctor in a junior grade, you won't be earning great money, and might start to wonder when you're ever going to be able to stop borrowing money from the bank or your parents. You can feel alienated from your colleagues, who are single and childless, and might think that you're never going to make it to the top. There are pros and cons to either way, and it's just a matter of finding out what's right for you, and your family.

> If you have all your kids while you're junior, then at least once you get to apply for your first proper job [as a consultant,] you can say to them, 'Well I've had my family, I won't be having any more …' I know it doesn't matter, well it shouldn't matter, or make any difference, but it does … Imagine if you were the person interviewing you
>
> *ST A&E*

Well, we've got two girls, and now they're a bit older, things have settled down … Part of me would really like another one, but then it's so nice to be able to go out, and not have to take the kitchen sink with me … If you have another one, there's all the stuff like transportation, and holidays … My husband said 'well, if you can guarantee that it's a boy, then yes!'

Consultant physician

When planning another pregnancy, remember that you need to be earning your normal salary during the maternity pay calculation period, as this will determine what maternity pay you receive (see Chapter 8).

Bear this in mind if you have taken a long period of maternity leave, and you want to have your children close together, or if you are working part time and earning a miserable salary.

We wanted a gap of about two and a half years between them … And in fact I'm pregnant again now! But this is definitely the last; this pregnancy was not exactly planned … It's roughly the same time interval again; I didn't want a big gap between them.

Consultant physician

As a junior, there are certain times when it can be more stressful to have a baby; if you're in run through training, and guaranteed a job for the next few years, you can feel more secure about taking time out, and trying to apply for a flexible training post on your return, if that's what you want to do. If you're coming to the end of a training programme, and would be reapplying for jobs at the same time as going off on leave, or on your return from maternity leave, then it might be wise to hold off until the future looks more certain. There will be certain times in your career when you're applying for competitive jobs, against other excellent candidates, and you might not feel confident to turn up to the interview 8 months pregnant (but see Chapter 1 for more information). It will depend on how you feel about it, how competitive your chosen field is, and how long your training is.

I planned both my children so I had them during my research … My second child, his due date was the deadline for my PhD … It was great, it made me really focused on finishing it. I remember kneeling down at the computer, two days before he was due, trying to finish it … My husband went with me to help me hand in the thesis, it was so huge I couldn't carry it!

Consultant dermatologist

I planned my children with careful reference to the BMA guidelines on maternity pay … And why not? I would say that you need to be careful; you need to make sure you know what you're entitled to. It's as if the information is some kind of secret, they keep it that way, but why shouldn't we try and plan our families like that?

GP

Chapter 18

Now we are six ... Watching your children grow

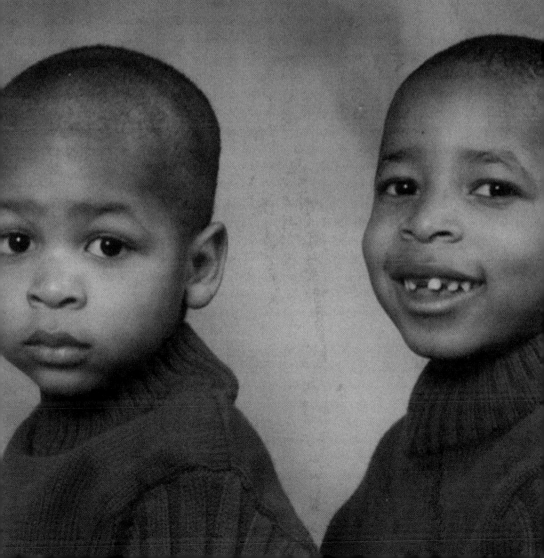

It gets harder as they get older … When they're young, it's all about us wanting to be with them, but as they get older they need you more … There's sport, and clubs, and projects … That's not the time to be thinking 'Right, I'll go full time now,' because nobody's interested in your kids as much as you are, and they want you to be there … You'll feel the pinch later on, [if you don't spend time with them then.]

Consultant renal physician

If the thought of choosing childcare for your baby brought you out in a rash, then wait until you have to get them into a school. Whether you choose private education, or state education, there are new hurdles to jump, and a new level of multitasking to aspire to. Childcare can be more complicated, as you have to get them to school and home again, and the summer holidays can stretch on for ever. Some schools have breakfast clubs, and after school activities, but you might still need to arrange school drop off and pick up, perhaps sharing the school run with other mums and taking it in turns to look after each others children after school, or finding a childminder who can look after them until you get home from work; see Chapter 14 for more information on childcare options.

When my son started nursery school, they wanted him to do a week of 'settling in,' just two hours a day … He'd been at full time nursery until then, and it was really difficult to arrange; I had to take a week of annual leave.

Consultant dermatologist

Sabbaticals

Both hospital doctors and GPs may be entitled to a sabbatical at some point in their career, to take a break from work for personal reasons, and return with new skills and experiences.

Sabbatical leave is usually paid leave of a short-term nature, up to a maximum of 6 months duration.

You are normally required to have a certain amount of service, i.e. be at the level of consultant or GP, but it's worth finding out about sabbaticals from your HR department; as a GP, any entitlement should be laid out in your contract.

Don't panic though, because help is at hand. Many schools provide activities before and after the 'normal' school day, allowing you to drop them off early and collect them later. Some schools will also offer play schemes, which run during the holidays. You may be able to use the 'breakfast club' first thing in the morning (often from 8 a.m.) and the after school activities (such as art, music, or sport) until 6 p.m. These services are not only based in the school grounds, but might also take advantage of local youth clubs, community centres or nurseries, and the staff may be teachers or local child-minders and voluntary groups. If school holidays are tricky to arrange, then you might find that willing grandparents or other relatives are only too pleased to help out. The most important thing to remember, if you can't arrange any help, is to get in early with organizing your annual leave.

> In the school holidays, she goes to the child minder, but it's the fact that if there's more than one of [your colleagues] that wants the school holidays, then you're juggling the dates … Half term is only a week, so you can have two people trying to both get the week off, and with summer holidays, it's a matter of who gets in first … But the summer holiday is the real issue … I try and take three of the summer weeks off, but then there's still a month in between, which to her seems an eternity… She's still dropped off at the child minders at 8 am, and collected at 6 pm in the evenings.

Consultant geriatrician

> What I tend to do [in the summer holidays], is I take two weeks off, my ex-partner takes two weeks off, then there's two sets of grandparents to cover the other two weeks.

Consultant physician

With all these different things going on, there's no need to feel guilty that you're 'dispensing' your children to third parties; remember when you were packed off to your grandparents for 2 weeks? Never in a million years did I imagine that my parents might feel guilty; why should they, when I was spending 2 weeks driving my grandparents potty and strangling my cousins, playing monopoly for days on end in a caravan in the rain, eating too many sweets, and loving every minute of it? Holidays aside, you can still feel bad about not being there to collect your child from the school gates during term time.

> At my son's school, they don't call it 'home time' at the end of the day … They call it 'mummy time!' It's awful, because I'm not always there to get him.

ST general practice

School holidays

....

The local educational authority decides on the dates of the school holidays. In general, state schools in the UK have 6 weeks off for summer, then 2 weeks at Christmas and at Easter. Half-term falls, well, half way, and is a week.

Contact your Local Authority or Children's Information Service for further information on kid's clubs, holiday clubs, etc.

If you want to book time off, you'll have to plan it with your colleagues who also have children; everyone may end up trying to get the time off at once.

Private schools often have different start and finish dates for the holidays, and may have longer or shorter holidays, which can be tricky if you have children of different ages at different schools.

He finishes school at 3.15pm. They have a breakfast club at 8.30, and then I have a childminder picks him up on my long days … On Thursday I do a half day and I can pick him up … Holidays are a mixture of us taking leave, and sending him off to parents, and a childminder … I worried that going from nursery to school would be a big problem, but I struck lucky with finding a good childminder.

Consultant renal physician

You may find that the Working Tax Credit (see Chapter 19) childcare element is available for some types of school-based childcare.

If your child has special needs

Contact a Family is a voluntary organization that provides support and information for families with disabled children. The helpline (0808 808 3555) may be able to put you in touch with other local families.

Contact your local Social Services Departments for information on short breaks, and play and leisure services for older disabled children.

One thing that just won't go away is the problem of sickness. Although they are (hopefully) poorly less often once they get to school, there will still be times when you have to phone in at the last minute. If the Calpol magic won't work, then you just have to remember that anyone else who is also a parent will understand what you're going through.

It's a huge, huge pressure … And I'm fortunate that she's not a sickly child. But occasionally, I'm sure she's gone to school on days that if I didn't work, she would have stayed at home … Not when she's been 'ill ill,' but on days when most children just want to curl up on the sofa, she's been pushed out the door with calpol.

Consultant geriatrician

Just like you did when your first baby was born, you need to find a new balance to life, and decide what matters and what doesn't. Your house will probably be clean again one day, and your kids aren't really bothered if their clothes are ironed or not.

If you can afford a cleaner, then why not invest in one; if you can't afford it, learn to look beyond the chaos.

> Having a good cleaner makes such a difference … You have to rationalize what is important, and what's not important… Anybody can cook, and clean, and iron, but you're the only person that can do their physics homework! So you make sure that you're there, and if their clothes are a bit grubby … Well, they get over it!'
>
> *Consultant surgeon*

> I've just had two weeks annual leave because the nanny was away, and you do all the things for them [the kids], you think 'Oh wow, this is really great, I've ironed all their clothes…' But then five minutes later you have to do it all again! If you try and do all the cooking, the cleaning, the ironing, because you think that's what it means to be a good mother … Well, it's absolute doo-doo.
>
> *Consultant surgeon*

Desperate housewives

- If you can afford a cleaner, even if it's just once a fortnight, go for it: £15 a fortnight could make a real difference to your quality of spare time with your kids.
- To find a good local cleaner, ask around friends and neighbours; you can find small ads in the papers and in shops, but a personal recommendation is much better.
- Some cleaners will do ironing as well.
- Look online or in the phone book for ironing services; some are surprisingly cheap, and you can leave a bag of ironing for a set fee.
- Cooking in bulk and freezing portions saves time and energy.
- Supermarket home delivery services can be fantastic, even if you just use it for the basics. You can often get free delivery if you choose certain times or days.
- Life's really too short to worry about these things.
- Finding a husband that's housetrained and cooks? Priceless.

I felt like I should be able to do some 'wife' things, knitting and sewing. Everyone said to me, 'Oh, you're no good, you couldn't possibly knit anything,' So I chose a pattern when I was pregnant, for a three year old child, and I slaved over it, and I completed it in eighteen months …!

Professor of Medicine

Whenever I feel guilty, I stop and remind myself why I'm doing what I do. I could have given up work once I had a child, and spent all my spare time with her. I could have taken her to school every day, and been there to collect her, and spent my evenings with her. But how would she feel when she was older? How would I ever persuade her that an education is important, and it's great to find a career you love and work hard at it, when I had given up? Every person is different, and I'm not for one minute suggesting that women who don't return to work have done the wrong thing. But for me, personally, I feel so lucky to be a doctor and a mum.

Our parents both worked full time [when we were growing up], and we always had a nanny or au pair, and my grandma helped out … And we had incredibly good neighbours; their mum didn't work and was always around. Our dad was home by six or six thirty and mum would be home later, about seven or eight … She'd often eat separately from us. But we always had six weeks of family holidays a year and we used to go abroad. I think I always thought I wanted to be a doctor, from quite early on, but our parents did try to put us off. It didn't work, as I am now a registrar in respiratory and ICU. My baby is six months old now, and I've gone back to work full-time this week. I'm doing research, but also doing clinical [ITU] on calls. In terms of childcare, it's excellent; the girl from the family next door [when we were growing up] is exactly the same age as me, and has a baby, so we share a nanny who is fantastic. We drop him off in the morning, and pick him up in the evening. The real problem is when I'm on call, and my husband [also a doctor] leaves for work before the nanny starts … But my friend is happy to let him stay overnight … And if the baby is sick, the nanny doesn't mind, she'll still look after him.

Susannah—Daughter of Professor Parveen Kumar

I do have my moments of doubt; the times when you just want to curl up on the sofa, but you've got a presentation to prepare; when the house looks like it's been burgled but it hasn't, and when my daughter points to the laptop and says 'mummy' when I'm trying to play with her. But all these things have to be balanced out with the days you get to spend with them, the fantastic family times, and the feeling you get inside when they come and plant a big kiss on your cheek by surprise.

My daughter thinks I work too hard … She doesn't want to be a doctor; she's decided to teach instead.

GP

I don't know if my mum being a doctor influenced my decision, but I suppose it did ... I do remember that if mum was working late, we sometimes had to go to the hospital ... She was a consultant radiologist, and it was always really exciting, she worked in this huge dark room, with loads of piles of stuff, films and notes, and x rays on the screens.

ST3 *medicine*

Reference

Department for Education and Skills (2006) *Looking for Childcare? A Surestart guide to help you make the right choices*. DfES Publications, Nottingham. www.surestart.gov.uk/aboutsurestart/parents/lookingforchildcare

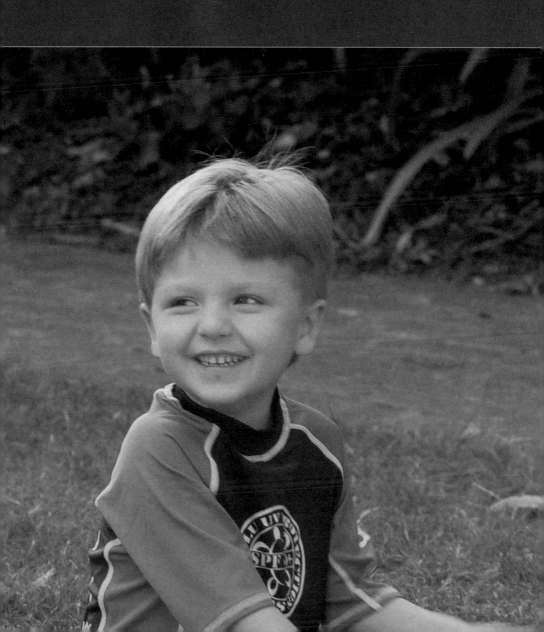

Chapter 19

Money matters

I got no maternity pay, nothing. All I get at the moment is child benefit … We're waiting for child tax credit; initially my forms were discarded, so we had to reapply … It's taking ages

FY1 doctor

- Maternity pay: see Chapter 8
- Paternity pay: see Chapter 16

Pensions

During the full pay period of maternity leave, contributions are payable on full pay. Once you are on reduced pay, your contributions are payable on the actual amount of pensionable pay you receive. Once you are on unpaid maternity leave, your contributions continue to be payable at the rate that applied during your reduced pay maternity leave.

During paid ordinary or additional maternity leave, your pension contribution should be calculated as if you were working normally.

When you are on unpaid maternity leave, your employer continues to pay contributions as if no reduction in pay had occurred.

If you don't return to work after your maternity leave, you must be given the opportunity to extend your pensionable service to take account of the statutory maternity pay. Contact your Human Resources department (or the BMA if you are a member) for more detailed advice on your pension.

Free prescriptions

Prescriptions are free for you while you are pregnant, and for the first 12 months after the baby is born. Your child will get free prescriptions until they are 16.

To claim for free prescriptions, you need to ask your doctor or midwife for form FW8, and send it to your primary care trust (in Northern Ireland ask for form HC11A, then send it to the Central Services Agency).

You will then be sent an Exemption Certificate, which is valid until 12 months after birth.

If you forgot to claim while you were pregnant, you can still claim after your baby is born; fill in form A in leaflet P11 NHS Prescriptions (in Northern Ireland HC11 Help with Health Costs), which you can either get from your doctor's surgery or Jobcentre Plus.

Free dental treatment

This is also free while you are pregnant, and for the first 12 months after your baby is born. You use the same exemption certificate, or tick a box on the form that the dentist gives you.

My partner is a full-time house-wife; I couldn't do it without him ... He can't claim any benefits, because he's not a UK resident ... But we get by.

FY1 doctor

Child Tax Credit

This is a payment for families with children. You can claim it if you are responsible for at least one child. You don't have to be working to claim it. It is to support:

1. A child until 1 September after their 16th birthday.
2. A teenager in full-time education aged 16–18.
3. A teenager who is aged 16 or 17, is not working or in full-time education, but has signed on with the Careers Service or Connexions Service, is not claiming their own income support or tax credits, and is not in prison (or is serving a sentence of less than 4 months).

You can get Child Tax Credit on top of Child Benefit and Working Tax Credit.

For information on how much you can claim, you need the leaflet from the Inland Revenue entitled *Child Tax Credit and Working Tax Credit—An introduction* (WTC1). The amount varies from about £2000 a year if you are not working, to about £200 a year if you have a joint income of £55 000. In general, you are paid more with every child you have, and more for children under the age of 1.

It is paid weekly or monthly, into a bank or building society account, or post office account.

Working Tax Credit

These tax credits are to top up the earnings of people on low incomes. There are extra amounts if you have a disability or if you have 'qualifying childcare' costs (see Chapter 14).

You can claim Working Tax Credit if you are responsible for a child or young person and work at least 16 hours a week.

It is paid on top of Child Tax Credit.

The amounts vary between about £5000 if you have one child and an annual joint income of £5000, to about £200 a year if you have a joint annual income of £55 000.

The childcare element within working tax credit

You may be able to get extra help with the costs of 'registered' or 'approved' childcare (see Chapter 14). You must be working at least 16 hours per week. This element is worth up to 70p in tax credit for every £1 a week you spend on childcare. It is limited to a certain amount, and there are maximum amounts you can claim; see the website for the most up to date details.

The childcare element of Working Tax Credit is paid directly to the main carer in the family.

Child Benefit

This is a tax-free benefit to help with the cost of caring for a child. You get child benefit for each child, up to the age of 16. You need to have lived in the UK for at least 6 months. It is paid to the mother, or the person responsible for the child.

For your first child, you get £18.10 per week, and for each extra child you get £12.10 per week.

Use the website http://www.direct.gov.uk to access the most up to date information on benefits available

If you were given a Bounty pack when you had your baby in hospital, you'll find a claim form inside. Otherwise you can get a form from your Jobcentre Plus, or post office (also from the General Registrars office in Northern Ireland).

Once you have filled in the forms, send them with your child's birth certificate to the Child Benefit Centre (child benefit office in Northern Ireland). You will get the birth certificate back, but it may take a while.

You can apply for child benefit online at http://esd.dwp.gov.uk/dwp/index.jsp

Child benefit is normally paid directly into your bank account, every 4 weeks in arrears. Single parents and families on low incomes can arrange for it to be paid weekly.

Make sure you start to claim child benefit within 3 months of your baby's birth, otherwise you will lose money.

If you choose to stay at home to look after your child, Child Benefit can help to protect your State Retirement Pension. You automatically get 'Home Responsibilities Protection' for every year that you get child benefit, but don't pay enough National Insurance to count towards the basic pension.

For queries about things that may affect the amount of child benefit paid: http://www.hmrc.gov.uk/childbenefit (Helpline 0845 302 1444, in Northern Ireland 0845 603 2000).

Child Trust Fund

Children born on or after 1 September 2002 are all given a £250 voucher to start a savings and investment account. The voucher belongs to the child, and they can't have it until they're 18.

You have a period of grace to choose a Child Trust Fund (CTF) account, but if you're normal, i.e. completely disorganized, the deadline may come and go. If that happens, the government will kindly invest your money for you.

People can make regular or one-off donations to the account; go the website http://www.childtrustfund.gov.uk for more information.

Student loans

Putting your student loan on hold:
If your gross monthly income is less than £2034 (2007), you are eligible to apply for deferment of your student loan. You need to ask for and complete form R15, and send it back with your last 3 months pay slips. If you don't have your pay slips, you can enclose a signed and dated letter from your employer on headed paper, confirming gross income for each of the last three calendar months.

If your application is approved, your student loan will be deferred for 12 months (but will still accrue interest).

You can reapply for further deferment after 12 months.

- Student Loans Company 0870 606 0704

General Medical Council (GMC) membership

If your forecasted gross annual income, from all worldwide sources, is less than £19 700, you are entitled to a 50% reduction in your annual fee (currently £290). To find the form (you need to fill it out and sign it) go to the website http://www.gmc-uk.org. The discount cannot be applied retrospectively.

About 8 weeks before your next registration payment is due, the GMC will write to ask whether you predict your next year's earnings to be below the threshold too. If you miss this opportunity to let them know, it may be too late, so don't put it in the recycling or line the hamster's cage with it.

If your income increases, you need to let the GMC know immediately, in writing, and send payment of £145.

BMA membership

If you are on maternity leave for the membership year, or if you earn less than £8620 from medical practice during the membership year, you can claim a reduction in fees under the 'temporary retirement' category.

Current rates are about £140 per year: http://www.bma.org.uk/ap.nsf/Content/subscriptionrates

Medical defence organizations

Contact your medical defence organization as soon as you know you are going on maternity leave; your fee for the time you are off may be reduced. Let them know if you are returning to the same job, at the same hours.

You should still be covered for 'Good Samaritan' acts: At 39 weeks gestation on a hot day, this is more likely to involve telling someone that they've got spinach in their front teeth, as opposed to doing cardiac compressions at a rate of 100 per minute.

Financial help if your child has special needs

You can apply for Direct Payments, to help with the costs of childcare. These are cash payments from your local authority, to help you buy your own support or care. Call 0845 602 2260 for the information leaflet, *A Parent's Guide to Direct Payments*.

Your Child Tax Credit may include additional payments for disabled children. You may also get extra help with childcare costs through Working Tax Credit. Call 0845 300 3900 for further advice, or for a claim form.

Contact your local Childrens' Information Service (CIS) for more information on local arrangements to help with the cost of caring for a disabled child.

Are babies expensive?

Whereas rolling around in mud and playing with their own toes comes cheap, there are some extra costs associated with having a baby. Don't think that you need to buy a new pine suite for the nursery if you're broke, as many things have a very short 'shelf-life' (such as Moses baskets and baby clothes) and can be begged or borrowed from neighbours, friends, and family. It's easy to feel like a negligent parent if your pram is second hand, or you don't buy a full compliment of 'Baby Einstein' DVDs, but babies really don't care, they just want happy parents. If you bottle feed, you'll need to buy some equipment, and most parents need a pram and a car seat. Nappies cost different amounts depending on whether you use cloth nappies or disposable (see below).

Supermarkets are great for cheap clothes (the amount you spend on an outfit is inversely proportional to the amount of time it will fit the baby before it's too small) and once you start weaning, it's cheaper to cook your own food at home and save 'organic biodegradable alfalfa' foods for times when you're out and about.

How much do nappies cost?

Disposable nappies

Newborn babies may need their nappy changing every couple of hours, day and night, but as your baby grows they need their nappy changed less often; a toddler may, on average, need their nappy changing about eight times a day.

Popular brand nappies are cheaper if bought in bulk. All nappies get more expensive as they go up in size, i.e. as your baby grows. The Eco-disposable nappies tend to be more expensive than normal disposables. A large pack (46) of popular brand nappies for a toddler costs about £9. For older babies, a large pack (20) of trainer pull-up pants costs about £5.

Re-useable nappies

Remember—you can use the nappies for all your children if you have more than one baby. You can buy second-hand nappies, which you can wash above 60° before use, from internet sites such as e-bay (http://www.ebay.co.uk).

Some councils encourage using cloth nappies by offering money off laundering services.

- All-in-one shaped nappy, about £12 each.
- Shaped two-piece nappy, about £8–12 each.
- Pre-folded nappy (need to use with a waterproof cover, £5–8 each) £1–4 each.
- Terry nappy, about £1–2 each.
- Liners cost £2 for a paper roll of 100, or £1–2 each if made of fleece.
  You probably need about 24 nappies for a newborn, plus about five waterproof covers.

For more information, contact the Cloth Nappy Campaign on 01245 437318 or go to http://www.essexcc.gov.uk/nappies/.

References

Department for Education and Skills. (2006) *Looking for Childcare? A Surestart guide to help you make the right choices*. DfES Publications, Nottingham. www.surestart.gov.uk/aboutsurestart/parents/lookingforchildcare
Department of Health (2004) *Birth to Five*. Department of Health Publications, London.

Chapter 20

Do you still wish you'd been a lawyer?

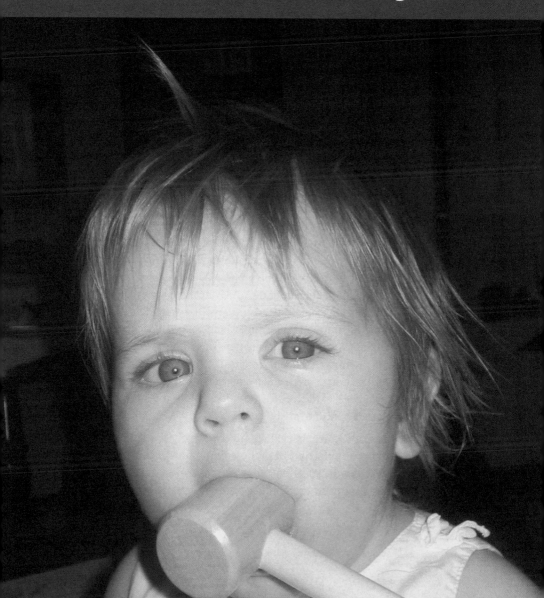

> Can you think of any other career where you can take a couple of years off, then just waltz back in at exactly the same level you left at, with the same pay as your colleagues? We are incredibly lucky in the NHS.
>
> ST haematology

We should all thank our lucky stars that we didn't choose law, or apply for a job in the city as a capitalist. Whereas it would be nice to earn half a million pounds a year, when it comes to pregnancy and family life, us doctors are luckier than you might think. Ballerinas, trapeze artists, air stewardesses, …; there are many jobs where being 8 months pregnant must be physically incompatible with doing your work. Some women are not allowed to work after a certain point in their pregnancy, such as pilots. Doctors, however, are not only allowed to become pregnant, but can continue working until the first stage of labour. Praise the day that you decided not to become a magician's assistant on a cruise ship; pregnant women are prohibited from working at sea after 28 weeks gestation. We are entitled to time off during our pregnancy for antenatal care, and we receive sick pay if we are unwell. In some countries, such as Denmark, women are only entitled to full sick pay during pregnancy if the illness is unrelated to pregnancy. Doctors can take a year of leave, then return to the same job either full time, or if funding is available, part time. We may struggle to breastfeed and work but it is possible, and unlike women working in a merchant bank, we might even have access to electronic breast pumps and storage facilities for our milk. Being a pregnant doctor might not be an easy ride at times, but for most female medics who choose to have a family; things work out alright in the end. A browse of the case studies in the Equal Opportunities Commission's booklet *Pregnancy and Maternity; your rights* (2006) make you feel relieved if you're still not convinced:

Until 1990, the armed forces had a policy of simply dismissing servicewomen who were pregnant. Nowadays, women receive compensation, based on the likelihood that they would have returned to work. Current policy at the Ministry of Defence states that any woman returning to work after having a baby must be expected to fulfil their full range of duties. In *Williams vs MOD* (2003 Employment Appeal Tribunal), Mrs Williams, a flight-lieutenant in the RAF, wanted to breastfeed her baby on her return to work, following maternity leave. The MOD required that she should be able to undertake her full range of duties, and would not be able to do so; the only other option offered was to take unpaid 'occupational maternity absence' until she was able to return to full duties; Mrs Williams resigned.

When you're frustrated, tired, and fed up, spare a thought for those women who, despite having made it to the top in a male-dominated profession, are unable to find a balance between work and family.

> Court is, by its nature, very difficult if you've got a child that's sick … If you don't turn up, then the whole thing has to be cancelled; the Judge's time is wasted, the jury's time is wasted, it has enormous financial consequences. So it is possible to work, but the only way to

do it is full time, to have very full on child care, and to be prepared not to see your kids for, well, weeks at a time. Friends of mine who are very ambitious, and are working, have a day nanny, a night nanny, and sometimes even a weekend nanny as well! Also, I know that junior doctors have the problem of being moved around the country, but at least you know where you're going to be for a few months ... We quite often don't know where we're going to be the next day! I practised for [about eight years] then I stopped when I had my third child. With my second child, I was in court until the day before he was born, then I had to return to work five weeks after he was born, because the trial was due to happen then; we applied to delay it by three weeks, but that was rejected. I didn't work Wednesday and Friday afternoons [for a few months], then I went back full time for the rest of the year, because that's how long the trial took. For some areas it's easier, for example in civil law, where there aren't so many trials, but in criminal law [where I worked], it's just difficult. I don't bear a grievance about it, because after all I'm the one who decided that I wanted to have children and to spend time with my children, so I could work if I wanted to. I suppose in the same way that some doctors side-step into general practice, some women who were in independent practice [before having children] either go and work for a company, or more commonly, work for the government, where things are much more child friendly. In terms of going back in the future ... Well; I think I've gone a bit chicken, because being in court is very nerve wracking ... And I don't know whether I could actually give enough of my time to it, my evening preparation, and the implications of someone going to prison if we lost the next day; I wouldn't want to feel that I hadn't actually prepared as well as I could have ... It's not an issue of competence; it's an issue of time.

Barrister

Once a doctor has given birth, not only does she have the right to return to her original post, but she might have the option of working part time, if that's what she chooses to do. It can be a bit of a pain sorting out the paperwork and making a few phone calls, but it won't be seen as anything unusual, to request that you spend more time with your young family. It was a different story in 2005 for Jessica Starmer, a 26-year-old pilot for British Airways, who ended up taking her employers to court for sex discrimination, after they rejected her plea to work at 50% in order to spend more time with her daughter. Maybe you think it's ridiculous that a pilot can work part time; maybe you think it's ridiculous that a surgeon can work part time; but if doctors do end up working at less than full time, it's generally accepted by their colleagues that they can still do their job properly.

You either come back and work from half six in the morning, 'til five, five days a week, or you don't come back ... Women do come back [after having a baby], but if you do, you come back properly, and you have a nanny ... Banks are highly competitive, so if I have to say to my client 'Look, I'm going to be off for six months, then I'll be back,' it's no good, they'll probably go elsewhere ... Clients want continuity.

Director (sales), Investment Bank

If you're still feeling terrible because your pregnant legs swell up on ward rounds, your child calls the nanny 'mummy', or your colleagues forget to invite you to the evening drinks because you're part time, then at least as a doctor you shouldn't be damned on moral grounds, for having had sex in the first place. Thanks goodness you're not a teacher: *O'Neill vs Governors of Thomas More RCVA Bedfordshire CC* (1996 Industrial Relations Law Report) is the case of a religious studies teacher at a Roman Catholic voluntary-aided school. She became pregnant by a Roman Catholic priest, who was known locally and in the school. And she was prevented from returning to work after she'd had the baby because of the 'moral and social implications of her pregnancy!'

Having a bad day? Reasons for doctors to be cheerful

1. Even if you work in a speciality where there are risks, such as radiology, you will be allowed to work, doing most of your normal duties, until the end of your pregnancy.
2. If you are sick during your pregnancy, you will get sick pay.
3. You may even get maternity pay.
4. On your return, you can go back at the same level, to the same job.
5. It is possible to breastfeed your baby on your return to work as a doctor.
6. You may have the option of part-time working, if you want it.
7. Even if you work less than full time, you will still be advancing your career.

In any industry, there's bound to be a bit of good old office tension when the work-load is high, but you have to leave on time to collect 'Little Johnny' from nursery. There's no easy answer to this, and in fairness, before I had a child I just had no idea what life would be like afterwards. You can't expect your colleagues to understand about kids, and life as a parent will often seem alien to them.

Obviously, our industry [women's magazines, publishing] is very child-friendly, because it's run by women. But what frustrates me, and my friends who are childless, is the treatment that these mums are getting ... I totally agree that mums have rights, but I've got many friends who've missed out on jobs, and women with kids have got them … Whereas my friends would have done Monday to Friday, nine'til six or seven if that's what was required on deadline day, but the job goes to a mother, who works four days a week, leaves at four o'clock … When you want to have an urgent meeting you can't, because they're never there, and you're the one who's left to pick up the mess. [If I had a baby], I don't know how I'd do my job … I'd be allowed to, but the people around me would have to make up the shortfall … They'd say, with open arms, come back and work four days a week. It's an industry that's so accepting of mothers … But I guarantee if you've got a colleague who's got a child; your workload will be doubled.

Celebrity Editor

We have fantastic jobs. We are privileged to share in the lives of our patients. If planning your first pregnancy is giving you palpitations, or if your nursery calls social services because you're late to collect (again), just relax, and remember that we are, all things considered, all right.

Looking back, I think I've been really lucky, I've landed on my feet … A lot of anxiety for nothing. You have these little crises every now and again, it's only natural, but look, what other job allows you to do this … Progress and train, but still spend time with your children?

Consultant physician

Reference

Equal Opportunities Commission (2006) *Pregnancy and Maternity; your rights*. Equal Opportunities Commission, London.

Frequently asked questions

Can I have a baby at any stage in my career?

> Once I was a consultant, the pressure to finish my training wasn't there ... so I took a whole year off, because I could! With my previous pregnancy, there had been a bulge of trainees trying to get through ... I went back part time, and it worked out very well ... one of my colleagues wanted to drop trauma, and I only wanted to do trauma, so the flexible careers scheme supported me very well.
>
> *Consultant trauma surgeon*

There's no right or wrong answer to this, and there is never a 'right' time! There are things you might want to take into account, like how long your training is, whether you can guarantee a part-time post in your speciality, what your partner does and how far through his training he is, as well as money issues. Women have children at all stages of a medical career; before they apply to medical school, or when they are a consultant or GP, and what's right for one family is not necessarily right for you. Whenever you decide to do it, you'll have to accept that you need to compromise in one aspect of your life or another; at the very least, even if you're going back full time, you'll need to take some time off for maternity leave. The main thing is to try not to get too stressed about the 'when' and just do it when it feels right.

> I did surgery, then care of the elderly, when I was really pregnant ... I was so pregnant, that I had to take breaks and sit down during the ward rounds ... It was such a big deal then, but now I see doctors sitting down on beds and stuff all the time, but it was a big deal then because I was only 'the student.'
>
> *Medical student*

See Chapter 1 for more information and advice from other doctors.

> I'm not even sure I'm bothered about becoming a consultant ...
> I think I just wanted to prove that I could get a [training] number.
> So now, I've got my number, I'm ready to find a man who I can have a family with.
>
> *ST surgery*

Do I have to do my night shifts in late pregnancy?

This will depend on your health and the health of the baby. If a specific risk is identified involving your night shifts, then you don't have to do them. If you feel fine and want to carry on, there are certain things you can do to try and make things easier; ensure that you get some rest during the day, and have enough with you to eat and drink when the canteens are all shut. Discuss your options with occupational health, and your team if possible, once you know the rota for the latter part of your pregnancy.

I thought they [my colleagues] would have noticed that I was pregnant [at 14 weeks], but they hadn't ... I worked quite late, and did my on calls far too late, until about 28 weeks. As a consultant, they were from home, but it was for a whole week at a time, so I got disturbed at least once every night, for a week ... Then I agreed to teach on an ALS course, I was knackered, and then I had her the following week ... I wasn't ready for it.

Consultant physician

See Chapter 3 for more information.

I'm a GP partner and worried about telling my colleagues that I'm pregnant. Will they be re-imbursed for my maternity pay?

This depends on where you work, and who you work with. All GPs need to scrutinize the maternity rights section of their contract before signing it; maternity pay and leave varies from practice to practice. You may be entitled to 6 months full pay, or you may get nothing. You might have to pay for your own locum cover. In some areas, the Primary Care Trust re-imburses the practice with several thousand pounds a month, but in others it doesn't.

It's easy to say don't feel guilty; it's only natural, as the practice is essentially a small business. Remember that most people, especially those who have had children themselves, will understand, as will your male colleagues with families.

See Chapters 4 and 8 for more information and advice.

Is research a good time to have children?

I was doing research when I had the first one ... I was in a really busy surgical registrar job when I got pregnant, and then I had a research job for about 18 months ... So I had my baby, and went back to full time work [in research] when she was nine months old. I think research is a very good time to have children, especially when it's your first, and you're still learning [how to be a mum], learning what way suits you ... You'll get lots of advice, but actually what works for you is very variable.

Consultant surgeon

When hospital jobs involved working a one-in-three rota (or worse), research was definitely a good time to have kids; being pregnant and being a lab rat was much more relaxing than running around with the labour ward bleep. Your hours will be more 9–5 in most areas of research, and covering days of sickness (yourself or the children) may be easier than when you're meant to be running a ward round or doing Monday morning surgery. Depending on the type of project you're doing, you may or may not be able to go back part time once you've had a baby; you need to talk to your supervisor about this early on.

When I was doing my PhD I could take him to nursery and pick him up afterwards ... His mum was working full time [as a medical registrar], so I was really lucky that I could see him so much ... It's different now I'm back doing clinical work.

Male ST medicine

Some people have told me that it's easier to have your children while you're a medical student. Is this true?

If this is the right time for you, then you'll make it work. You might be a mature student, not wanting to wait until you're qualified, or you might have always wanted to have children when you were young. Maybe your pregnancy was a surprise; whatever your reasons, you have people around you to help make it work. At least you won't be on call as a junior doctor when you're heavily pregnant, and you won't spend the first half of your working life worrying about when and how to have children. You'll have emotional support available from your tutors, and you may be entitled to some financial help; but be prepared that you might end up struggling with money if your partner isn't earning. You'll need some time off from your studies too, and may end up in the year below all your current friends.

See Chapter 6 for more information and advice.

What do I do if I'm off sick during my pregnancy? Do I have to go on maternity leave early?

There are regulations in place to protect you and your baby, and any risks should be identified and reduced or eliminated. You cannot be dismissed because you are pregnant, or for reasons connected with your pregnancy or maternity leave.

My pregnancy markers went up, because of my hypertension ... So I got a false positive for Downs, and I had to have an amniocentesis. After the amnio, I was supposed to rest for seven days, because of the risk of miscarriage ... But the consultant called me at home, and was really angry. In the end they said to me 'Look, we know you're having problems, but we have a service to run,' so I had to say 'Fine, I'll give you notice now, but I'm going off sick. Then I ended up not being paid; once I started to inquire why, I made a fuss, they were bending over backwards, and the money was suddenly in my bank account.

ST paediatrics

If the risks to you and your baby cannot be removed, and alternative work cannot be offered to you, then you have to be suspended on full pay.

See Chapter 7 for more information on employment law.

Going off sick during your pregnancy can affect your maternity leave. In simple terms, if it is in the last month of your pregnancy (before you had planned to stop work), your maternity leave will have to start early. Sickness earlier on during the pregnancy should be treated as normal sick leave, and paid as such. Sickness unrelated to pregnancy in the last month will also be treated as normal sick leave, and will not affect your maternity leave.

See Chapter 8 for more detailed information on maternity leave for hospital doctors and GPs.

How much maternity leave and pay do hospital doctors get?

Refer to Chapter 8 for more detailed information on what you might be entitled to; maternity laws in the NHS are complex, and there is no single rule for everyone. The following is a very rough guide.

You are entitled to 26 weeks of Ordinary Maternity Leave (OML) plus 26 weeks of Additional Maternity Leave (AML).

You will be entitled to maternity pay if you have worked for 12 continuous months, either full or part time, and you intend to return to work for the NHS for a minimum of 3 months after your leave.

If you qualify, then you will get 8 weeks of full pay (less statutory maternity pay SMP or maternity allowance, MA). You will then get 18 weeks of half pay, plus any SMP or MA (as long as the total doesn't exceed your normal full pay).

> My reasons for going back early [after three months] are financial, as I've been in the system for less than twelve months, so my maternity leave is unpaid ... Also I've only got two years of training left, and I want to get it over with as soon as possible. My plan at the moment is to go back full time, and organize set days and on-call nights that I work ... Then I'm sitting my final anaesthetics exam in March or April, when the baby will be six months old.
>
> *ST anaesthetics*

How much maternity leave and pay do GPs get?

ST3 doctors (GP Registrars) are covered by the NHS scheme as outlined above during their hospital posts, and should be covered by them as an ST3.

Salaried GPs may be entitled to both paid and unpaid maternity leave, but their contract should outline their own individual entitlements.

GP partners will have their entitlements written into their contract.

> I got six months full pay ... But then, I did help to write the partnership agreement, which helps!
>
> *GP*

Should I go to antenatal classes? I am doctor after all ...

When you're pregnant and working full time, the last thing you want to do is go and be taught (again) about the different stages of labour, and watch a plastic dolly being shoved through a model of the pelvis. Even if you're an experienced obstetrician, you might find it helpful to go along, to meet other mums and have a tour of the wards if you're not having the baby at work.

The classes won't just deal with the physical facts of childbirth. The emotional aspect of childbirth is often explored, and simple relaxation techniques can be learned (even if you think drugs are more useful). You'll discuss breastfeeding, and how to cope in the early days; just don't tell anyone that you're a doctor, in case you get asked to do a quick demonstration of perineal massage.

Should I have my baby in the Trust that I work in?

> I walked onto labour ward, and the first person I met was the anaesthetic SHO, who had been on my ATLS course the previous week ... He just looked at me and said 'Oh no, no way, I'm phoning the consultant and telling him you're here ...' and I said 'Look, I might not want an epidural,' and he said 'I don't care, I'm telling him that you're here!'
>
> *Consultant surgeon*

Do you want your medical students to see you naked, and will you regret anything you happen to shout during labour? If you're not bothered, and you actually feel more comfortable in a familiar environment, then it might be fine having your baby where you work. You might find that as a local GP or a fellow hospital doctor, the team bend over backwards to make everything nice for you. Other women might prefer to remain anonymous, and not disclose that they're medical at all, whereas others might want to be a doctor, but a doctor away from people who know them.

> My friend, a GP reg, had just had a really terrible delivery, but the doctor [the obstetrics registrar] was really nice to her ... Then he went outside the room and looked at the notes, and she overheard him say 'God, she's only a bloody registrar, I thought she was a GP!'
>
> *GP*

After 10 years as a doctor, I still don't understand what a Health Visitor or community midwife does

Your community midwife is a midwife who looks after you and the baby from birth, until the baby is roughly between 10 and 28 days old. They should check the baby is feeding ok, give you help with breastfeeding, and check your perineum if you had stitches, or check your caesarian scar.

Health visitors are qualified nurses. They receive extra training in looking after people in the community. They should be able to offer advice about feeding, weaning, sleep problems and behavioural issues.

Both midwives and health visitors should be on the lookout for signs of postnatal depression, and should be able to refer you on for more specialised help if needed.

See Chapter 11 for more information.

How will I meet other new mums?

Unless you lock yourself in the house with your baby and don't go outside, you'll find that it's quite easy to meet new mums. You may have made some friends at antenatal classes, and your community midwife or health visitor can always introduce you to other mums in your area. Baby massage, swimming, and the playground are all great places to meet other people, and even if you're shy, you'll find that your children aren't, so they'll do the introductions for you! The National Childbirth Trust (NCT) can help introduce you to other working parents in your area, and if you start using a local nursery you'll find that you bump into the same people time and again.

See Chapter 11 for more advice on the early days.

Can I return to work part time?

> My reg went back full-time; she's got two little ones ... But now, I think the youngest is 22 months, she's really depressed, regretting what she's done, she feels like she's missed out ... But she wanted to get her training done.
>
> ST medicine

If you work part time, then your training will take longer and your pay will drop. But you will get the chance to balance work and family, and spend valuable time with your children. You need to have a job first, from which you apply to work part time. Most of the Royal Colleges have a flexible training adviser, who can give you advice and information on working flexibly in your chosen speciality.

> I think I'm going to work every morning at first; my mum and dad are going to help out. Then I get to be around for the afternoon, there won't be a day when I don't see the baby.
>
> ST general practice

You have no automatic right to return to work part time once you've had a baby. You can apply to work part time, and there may or may not be a job, or funding, for you. Part-time doctors in general practice work a certain number of sessions as agreed with the partners. Hospital doctors can work as a slot share where they are employed and paid as individuals (one training job, shared between two doctors, usually at 60%). A supernumerary post means that you are an 'extra' pair of hands. In a job share, each doctor does half the hours and gets half the pay.

I couldn't get a part-time job, so I had no option—go back full time or don't go back. So I gave up medicine, and now I teach music, I'm a private tutor.

Previous ST surgery

Most other medics will see you as a lucky doctor, who has the world at her feet. A few will see you as a worse doctor; they must be jealous.

Well, it's all this left wing bloody liberalism isn't it, forcing us to allow doctors to work part time. I mean, you can't be a proper doctor working two days a week. What a shame she had to just go and give up her career like that.

Consultant orthopaedic surgeon (said to a patient, who had just told the surgeon that his wife was a part-time GP)

Chapter 12 has more information on working part time.

Can I breastfeed and work full time?

Yes. If you want to do it, you can breastfeed your baby while you're doing full days, on calls, night shifts. It just takes a bit of organizing, some understanding from colleagues, and some equipment.

At [my hospital] I used to take the machine in to work with me … I used to go to the maternity wards to express … Normally they would give me a cubicle, but one time, they gave me this amazing room, I was like wow, where did this come from?! It was a beautiful double bedroom … When I was a student and expressing, my first firm back, I said to my consultant in front of everyone, all the other students, 'Look, I have a baby at home and I'm breastfeeding, do you have a room where I can express?' And she was really taken aback and said 'Well, nobody's ever asked me that before!' … But then it was all fine. I was really worried about saying it, it really played on my mind, like I had to just get it off my chest as soon as possible to check it was ok.

FY1 doctor

Some people, including health professionals, will tell you that you can't do it, because your milk supply will dry up. With the positive feedback mechanism in mind, remember that as long as you continue to express milk, and feed your baby when you're with them, your milk supply will be fine.

I spoke to the sister on SCBU, and they said they had a couple of bedrooms that I could use, if they were free. I had a breast pump, and they let me keep all the sterilizing stuff there … They were really helpful. So I used to go down and express in the middle of the day, you know, eating a sandwich and staring at pictures of my daughter ... They even let me freeze it and leave it there; I just took what I needed for the next day. I was really lucky, and the nurses got to know me and were great. I didn't tell my male colleagues where I was going, I just used to say 'Look, I need to go off for a while ...' I think they knew what I was doing, but we never talked about it.

Consultant physician

See Chapter 13 for more experiences of breastfeeding and working.

I'm terrified about my first day back after maternity leave. Any advice?

You'll feel less scared if you've managed to keep in touch during your leave, even if it's just popping in with the baby for a cup of tea every now and again. Make sure you sort out your child care well in advance, so you're not panicking about that, and make sure that your first day back isn't the first time you have to leave your baby all day. Check that your work clothes still fit you, and get everything ready the night before. If you have time, doing a dummy run to work a few days before can really help.

Don't panic. You're going to spend most of the day showing everyone pictures of your baby and talking about them. You'll probably be surprised how much you enjoy being back.

See Chapter 15 for more information.

What's the best type of childcare?

I work on the dialysis unit, and I've had to take him into work a few times ... The nurses on the ward help out and entertain him.

Consultant renal physician

Jimmy Choos or Clarks sensible shoes? Both will satisfy a need for footwear on a particular occasion, but different people have different needs. What is right for one family is wrong for another, and money, flexibility, and personal preferences all have to be taken into account, as well as the age of your child or children and their own needs and preferences. Chapter 14 attempts to decipher the different types of childcare available to you, with the pros and cons of each.

I took [my daughter] out of nursery for a couple of days a week, to be with me and the baby, but those days were a complete nightmare! She would run across the road when I was stuck there with the pram, or she'd want to ride her scooter, then decide after a while that she didn't, and I'd have to carry her, and the scooter, and push the pram ... But now, they're really good friends.

Consultant physician

How do I juggle work, small children, and a life outside medicine?

> It is true that the parents have to have a degree of happiness to make their children happy ... Other people may look at me and think I don't spend enough time with my kids, but I'm still their mum, and I'm the only mum they've got.
>
> *Consultant surgeon*

I've never got the hang of juggling oranges, but I suppose if I had enough practice I'd be really good. In the same way that you learn how to be a doctor, you'll learn new ways of getting out of the house on time, getting away from work on time to collect your kids, and maintaining a relationship with your partner. It sounds like a lot to ask, but with time you'll adapt.

> Work is no longer number one ... I was very focused as an SpR, I was a work orientated person, and having your family does make you think differently about things. You realize that you can't conquer Rome in a day, and there are things you just have to let go.
>
> *Consultant diabetologist*

There will always be some compromises to make; maybe your house looks like you've had a party in it, maybe you'll forget someone's birthday once in a while. As long as it's not your child's birthday, they'll get over it. Think back to the day when you were a house officer, with your lists of jobs, and remember that most of them got done, most of the time. You've had years of practice at multitasking, and you're probably fairly good at it by now.

> My son woke up at four o'clock in the morning, and he came looking for me in the study, not the bedroom ... He said he thought I lived there ... That really made me stop and think!
>
> *Consultant dermatologist*

See Chapter 15 for more ideas.

What do I do if my kids are sick and I've got an operating list or a full surgery?

> But you feel guilty, because even now, [my daughter] says to me, 'I have to be dying, don't I, to get a day off school ...' My husband and I are pretty tough ... I've had three days off in 14 years ... I was brought up that way. So I feel there's a pressure put on you, and there's no flexibility in the NHS. I'm sure, if your child was sick, and was in hospital, that people would make allowances, but that's what it is;

making allowances ... And there's a degree of resentment, especially from those who haven't got children. The ones who've got children, even the blokes, are very understanding ... The ones who don't, they are less understanding when your childcare goes awry; which it does, with the best will in the world: The nanny gets sick, or your child minders children get sick, and they can't take your kids in case it's something infectious ... And you are left then, well, with saying I have to look after my child. It is a pressure on you, and it doesn't go away.

Consultant physician

There's no easy answer to this one. There might be times, especially when your children are small, when they seem to be ill constantly; just getting over one thing (and giving it to you) then getting another thing straight away. At the end of the day, you have a commitment to your family, and a commitment to your patients, and different women will prioritize differently. A lot will depend on how sick your child is, whether you have childcare at home or at a nursery, and how flexible your partner is. In a junior post, or as a supernumerary doctor, it's easier to miss the odd day here and there without it seeming so disastrous, but if you're the consultant in charge things can be tricky.

My daughter hates having parents who are doctors ... she never gets a day off sick from school ... We give her calpol and send her on her way!

Consultant physician

Everyone's going on about the mums, but what about the medical dads?

When you hear about male [surgical] consultants with kids, they don't get to see them do they—they work late into the evening, and they're there first thing in the morning. I don't think they get to see their kids ... The plastic surgeons, part of the reason that put me off doing it, was that they'd ring them up even if they weren't on-call. They would say '... It's one of your patients, the flap's gone dusky, are you going to come in?' And nine times out of ten they would ... So you've got that in the back of your mind, that's what's expected of you ... But you couldn't do that if you were looking after a child ... I think that was part of the reason I decided against Plastics ... I can't make that kind of lifestyle choice.

ST surgery

Poor dads; after the baby's born, everyone seems to be fussing around the mum and the baby. The guy who contributed so enthusiastically at the point of conception has to go back to work, leading long ward rounds or seeing other people's kids all day in their surgery. Paternity leave is for 2 weeks (see Chapter 16 for more information), but after that very few male doctors work part time. If their partner is having a bad day, he may only be able to have a quick 2-minute conversation with her between patients, and he may come home one evening to find that his mother-in-law's moved into the house permanently. At least when the baby is small, and awake half the night, there's plenty of opportunity for nocturnal bonding; but come the toddler years, they might be fast asleep by the time he comes home from work, and waking up in the morning just as he leaves.

> Very early on, I had about a month or so where all my on calls were close together ... So I didn't really see him, or [my partner] ... He seemed to get a bit clingy then, but maybe that was natural at that age anyway. Now, I get up an hour or so early in the morning, just to spend time with him before I go to work ... He tends to wake up at about 5.30am anyway!
>
> *ST medicine*

> My children just had to put up with an absent father ... I was a registrar in orthopaedic surgery when they were small. But my life as a doctor has been incredible. I wouldn't have used my time in any way other than being a doctor.
>
> *Consultant orthopaedic and trauma surgeon*

Should I have all my children close together, to get things out of the way sooner?

> I've met a couple of really senior doctors who had a full four or five years off when they had their kids, then went back to work ... When I said 'Really?' they said 'Well yes, of course, why not?' As if it was the most normal thing in the world to do. It had really worked for them.
>
> *ST haematology*

Some couples decide to have small age gaps between their children, either due to mis-calculation, or because they want to get all the early years over sooner (nappies, sleep deprivation, goo on the wallpaper, etc.) Others decide to space their children out, enjoying the early years with each child in turn. The decision may be influenced by money, space at home, length of training paths or numerous other factors, but like everything else baby-related, the choice is yours. Different things suit different people. There are probably pros and cons to each, and Chapter 17 has more information.

Who invented long summer holidays? What am I supposed to do about childcare?

The dates of the school holidays are decided by the local education authority, or by the school itself if it's a private establishment. Most UK state schools have 6 weeks off for the summer.

If you're lucky, you may have parents who are able to help out, who will delight in having your kids for a couple of weeks. My parents would never have sat, in the pouring rain, while I went on the same roller coaster 25 times at Morecombe Pleasure Beach, but my grandparents seemed to enjoy it. Playing monopoly with my cousins and scoffing sweets for 2 weeks non-stop was heaven in those days; remember that you're doing your kids a favour too!

If you don't have the option of parents, you may be able to take some leave over the summer. Your childminder might be available for holidays (but some aren't) or there might be local holiday clubs and activities.

See Chapter 18 for more information and ideas.

Can I reduce any of my monthly outgoings when I'm on unpaid maternity leave?

There are ways to help your money go further; prescriptions for you and the baby are free, as is dental treatment. The leaflet GL23 Social security benefit rates is available from your Jobcentre Plus, outlining some benefits that may be available to you. You may be entitled to Child Tax Credit, which is a payment for families with children. You'll also be able to claim Child Benefit.

In terms of reducing your monthly outgoings, you may find that payments to the Student Loans Company, the General Medical Council, the British Medical Association and your medical defence organization can all be suspended or reduced; see Chapter 19 for more information.

Any final comments from the medical mums?

I've got a few patients who, over the years, always ask 'how's your daughter?' There's one patient, who's really quite demented and has just gone into a nursing home, but whenever I see her, she always remembers that I have a daughter and asks how she is!

Consultant geriatrician

The worst thing I did actually ... Was to take my sabbatical! Because I suddenly realized, and appreciated, what it was like to be with them all the time ... I realized all the things I miss out on ... It made me feel quite resentful about going back to work ... Who knows what the right balance is.

GP

I think that you're a better doctor if you've been through the experience and actually have to think about someone else before yourself. It makes you put a whole different perspective on the way you practice medicine ... I practice differently now to before I had her.

Consultant physician

The only things you can give your kids are your genes and a good education ... The rest is by the by, don't worry about the housework!

Consultant surgeon

It's a double-edged sword [being a doctor and being a mum] ... I remember my daughter having a bad headache, then I found out she had photophobia and neck stiffness ... My husband and I spent the night wondering what to do ... In the morning she saw a friend of ours, a consultant paediatrician, of course she was fine, but I wonder if we weren't both doctors we wouldn't have been so worried.

Consultant physician

You ask different questions [when you're a mum] ... If you see a young patient in casualty, and you know they've got a baby, you ask who's looking after the baby ... And you just have to see a sick child, and you burst into tears! It gets better as they get older, but it doesn't go away.

Consultant physician

He doesn't like going to [my husband's GP] surgery, he thinks it's boring there ... One day I collected him from the childminder at half six and had to take him back to the hospital, and he was in the car shouting 'No! Not the hospital!'

Consultant physician

The first [baby] I had when I was a year five SpR ... I was sitting my exit exam, and I wanted to have her after the exam ... I'd waited as long as I could in my training to have her. I didn't want to be taken less seriously, if I'd had her earlier on.

Consultant trauma and orthopaedic surgeon

A lot of the reason I changed to GP [from A&E], was to have children ... Five more years of doing nights, with kids, that would be ridiculous ... Now I do one a month! I can't imagine being as tired as I was ... I used to do, when I was a medical SHO, 26 days in a row ... I can't imagine doing that with a baby ... Some of that's changed, with shift patterns though.

ST general practice

I used to have these crises, and think 'Oh god, I'm so slow, I'm going to end up in a District General Hospital in the middle of nowhere doing MAU,' but here I am in [a big teaching hospital], doing what I want to do, and I've got my kids too ... You have to step back every now and again, and think wow, I'm really lucky.

Consultant renal physician

From the surgical side of things, my experience of people who have gone and got pregnant whilst they've been doing surgical training has been ... Predominantly negative. There was a girl I remember at X Hospital, who was pregnant with her first child, and I remember the comments that were made about her behind her back when we were in meetings and that, that she had 'Ruined her career, because she was having a child', and she was in her thirties!

ST urology

Forget being a doctor ... I'm on the lay websites on the internet looking up all my problems, the stuff I learnt in obs and gynae is irrelevant ... I'm learning so much from these random women on the web, stuff that actually matters, stuff I really want to know that the text books don't tell you. I was freaking out about having 'period pain' cramps for weeks until I read all the stuff about it ... It happens to so many women!

ST general practice

My National Childbirth Trust classes are two consecutive Saturdays ... And I'm absolutely dreading meeting a patient there! Potentially I could, it'd be awful.

GP

Even when [pregnant] people call, for advice about constipation, or advice on diet, I ask them to talk to the Health Visitor, as I don't really know the best advice, she's much better.

GP

There's a lot of stuff I don't know about, like positions in labour, and use of TENS, and I don't want to just go down a medical route ... I'm going to the NCT ... But I'm really anxious about becoming medicalised.

GP

I had lots of hyperemesis in pregnancy, and because I was working in a hospital [in India] away from my family, I didn't have any support ... So in fact I resigned from that job, because of the hours and everything ... My husband had gone to the UK at that time. I carried on, then in the second trimester my scan showed my cervix was a bit short ... I just thought that's it, I have to stop this. After [I had resigned] I did some exams, I did my part one obs and gynae and my PLAB ... And had some quiet time. Because I was planning to come to the UK to join my husband I had no intention of going back to that job.

ST obs and gynae

I went back after 12 weeks, and one of my patients said 'Oh, you've been on a long holiday ...' When I told her I'd had a baby, she said 'Well you did look rather fat!'

GP

I've had fairly patronizing comments from midwives all the way through ... But it's really interesting to find out what patients go through ... If I was a 'normal' patient, I'd come away from every appointment thinking 'Oh no, my baby's too small, I should rest, I've got to lie down, and drink lots of milk ...' And really, I'm not worried, but it winds me up!

GP

So I'm there at 2am doing fundoscopy on my pregnant wife because she's got a headache ... Sometimes it would be easier to not be a doctor.

ST medicine

Although I want to be a good doctor, I'm not as bothered as I am about being a good mum.

ST general practice

I would rather be a happy mum, working harder to balance my two precious worlds, than be a disgruntled mum, from having sacrificed my career.

ST psychiatry

I had my first daughter when I was an SpR, quite near the end of my specialist training. Before I got pregnant, I was working with another female reg, and one day we were chatting with a consultant in the department of psychological medicine [about having children] ...
She said, 'Well if I were you, I'd get broody! There simply isn't a right time, and you can spend forever putting it off, then find out that you're too old.'

Consultant physician

I put it off [being pregnant], because we were setting up the practice, so I waited until we had been there for some time.

GP

I remember in my interview for the surgical rotation, the panel saying 'Well we hope you're not planning on getting married or having any children soon!'

ST surgery

I was on call, and running around the hospital one evening, and I went to the loo and realised I was bleeding ... I knew I was pregnant, a few weeks, but I hadn't told anybody. I was so scared, and I remember going to the EPAU and finding one of the obs and gynae SHOs ... He took me into a side room, and he was so nice to me, he said 'Look, you really need to try and put your feet up, have a break,' because I couldn't stop crying ... But while he was talking to me, my bleep must have gone off about ten times in a few minutes, and I thought 'How the hell am I going to have a break?!' He knew I couldn't. I worked until the end of my shift, a few more hours, then went home. I didn't have a miscarriage, but I took a few days off. My husband rang my consultant, because I was too scared, and he couldn't have been nicer to me, he was so kind. He went out of his way to make sure everything was alright for me after that.

FY1 surgery

All the seniors were saying 'Hey, you should relax,' but when I was on with them, they wanted me to rush around and do the work for them!

ST medicine

I sat Membership [exams] when I was 24 weeks pregnant ... It was the practical part ... I was wearing a dress and a blazer that didn't do up if I put anything in the pockets, so I couldn't take my ophthalmoscope because it didn't fit in the pocket ... I was there in my exam trying to explain to the examiner why I didn't have it with me ... And I thought god what am I doing, telling him I'm fat?! What on earth does he think of me!

Consultant physician

I'll never forget the rolling of the eyes, when this poor SHO, who was six and a half months pregnant, had to sit down on a long ward round.

ST medicine

The empathy that you strike with a pregnant woman [in antenatal clinic], it's definitely increased—they feel like you know what they're going through.

Consultant diabetologist

It's definitely a good time to do it ... In GP-land people understand that you're a woman, you're going to want to have babies, it's more accepted. But I feel like I've screwed my practice really badly. They can't take on another registrar while I'm on maternity leave, because I have to have the option of returning before the 12 months is up, whatever I say now about definitely wanting to take 12 months ... So they lose all their funding and stuff, and they loose their registrar.

ST general practice

The patients were all just lovely [about the pregnancy] ... I think it's fair to say that they were part of it! It was very much 'their baby', and now, he's three, but they still ask 'how is he?' 'Is he at school yet? They were just delightful about it.

GP

I don't really know [whether to tell them I'm a doctor] ... I know that on the front page of my notes it says that my partner is a doctor ... But so far the only person to have picked up on that was the ultrasonographer, who had just given us a lecture on what the hypothalamus does ... And she was just mortified when she found out; she said 'Oh god, I can't believe I told you what the hypothalamus does ...' But actually at the time, we quite liked it, because we didn't know!

GP

They wanted to do a CT of my pelvis and I was in this [hospital] nightie and I had a pleading thing with a porter, saying 'Please let me walk,' and him saying 'Please let me take you in a chair,' and after about five minutes of this I got in the chair, then I had to be wheeled down these miles of corridors with everyone I knew seeing me, and saying 'Hi!', and me just feeling awful in this chair in this grubby little nightdress.

Consultant physician

One of my colleagues has just had three years off ... A total break from clinical work of at least two years, and she's finding it difficult, with her confidence ... I think that doing work gives you confidence, and

I would say that even during your maternity leave, you should try and go in, even just for the odd meeting, to keep in touch, to stop feeling so isolated.

GP

I came back to work full-time when my baby was four months old ... I didn't want to, but my mum said if I didn't go back then, I'd never go back. So she moved in with us, and she looks after him. I remember my breast milk stopping, and I thought 'Well that's it then, he doesn't need me any more ...' I really, really missed him.

ST rheumatology

Appendix 1

Useful contacts

Adoption and fostering

British Association for Adoption and Fostering
Saffron House
6–10 Kirby Street
London EC1N 8TS
Tel.: 020 7421 2600
http://www.baaf.org.uk

Government information—adoption and fostering
http://www.direct.gov.uk/en/Parents/AdoptionAndFostering/index.htm

Breastfeeding

Association of Breastfeeding Mothers
PO Box 207
Bridgwater
Somerset TA6 7YT
Counselling Hotline: 08444 122949 (9.30am–10.30pm)
General enquiries: 01278 459747

The Breastfeeding Network
PO Box 11126
Paisley PA2 8YB
Supporterline: 0870 900 8787

La Leche League
PO Box 29
West Bridgford
Nottingham NG2 7NP
Tel.: 0845 456 1855 (Mondays and Thursdays)
Tel.: 0845 120 2918 (24-hour helpline)

National Childbirth Trust Breastfeeding Line
Tel.: 0870 444 8708
7 days a week from 8am to 10pm

Childcare

4Children (formerly the Kids' Clubs Network)
City Reach
5 Greenwich View Place
London E14 9NN
Tel.: 020 7512 2100
Email: Info@4Children.org.uk
http://www.4children.org.uk

Childcare Approval Scheme
For checking on home-based child carers such as nannies.
Tel.: 0845 7678 111
http://www.childcareapprovalscheme.co.uk

Childcare Link—To contact your local Children's Information Service (CIS)
Tel.: 0800 2346 346
http://www.childcarelink.gov.uk

Children's Information Service (CIS)
See 'Childcare Link'.

Daycare Trust
(National childcare charity)
21 St. George's Road
London SE1 6ES
Tel.: 020 7840 3350
Email: info@daycaretrust.org.uk
http://www.daycaretrust.org.uk

National Childminding Association (NCMA)
Royal Court
81 Tweedy Road
Bromley
Kent BR1 1TG
Tel.: 0800 169 4486 (general information)
http://www.ncma.org.uk

National Day Nurseries Association (NDNA)
Unit 13
Pennine Business Park
Longbow Close
Bradley Road
Huddersfield HD2 1GN
Tel.: 0870 774 4244
http://www.ndna.org.uk

Ofsted (The Office for Standards in Education)
National Business Unit
3rd Floor
Royal Exchange Buildings
St Anne's Square
Manchester M2 7LA
0845 640 4040—Helpline

Tel.: 08456 40 40 40—Complaints about childcare providers (Mon to Fri 8am to 8pm)
http://www.ofsted.gov.uk

Pre-School Learning Alliance (PLA)
Tel.: 020 7697 2500
http://www.pre-school.org.uk

Professional Association of Nursery Nurses (PANN)
2 St James Court
Friars Gate
Derby DE1 1BT
Tel.: 01332 372 337—for an information pack on employing a nanny
Email: pann@pat.org.uk
http://www.pat.org.uk

Sure Start
Tel.: 0870 000 2288
http://www.surestart.gov.uk

Deaneries

Eastern Deanery
Postgraduate Medical & Dental Education
Block 3 Ida Darwin
Site Fulbourn Cambridge CB1 5EE
Tel.: 01223 884 822
http://www.easterndeanery.org

East Midlands Healthcare Workforce Deanery
University of Nottingham
Kings Meadow Campus
Lenton Lane
Nottingham NG7 2NA
North Office—Tel.: 0115 846 7102
South Office—Tel.: 0116 2952240
http://www.eastmidlandsdeanery.nhs.uk

Mersey Deanery
Regatta Place
Brunswick Business Park
Summers Road
Liverpool L3 4BL
Tel.: 0151 285 4722
http://www.merseydeanery.ac.uk

Kent, Surrey and Sussex Deanery
7 Bermondsy Street
London SE1 2DD
Tel.: 0207 415 3401
http://www.kssdeanery.ac.uk

London Deanery
Stewart House
32 Russell Square
London WC1B 5DN
Tel.: 020 7866 3100
http://www.londondeanery.ac.uk

Northern Deanery
Postgraduate Institute for Medicine and Dentistry
University of Newcastle
10–12 Framlington Place
Newcastle upon Tyne NE2 4AB
Tel.: 0191 222 8908
http://www.pimd.co.uk

Northern Ireland
NIMDTA
Beechill House
42 Beechill Road
Belfast BT8 7RL
Tel.: 028 9040 0000
http://www.nimdta.gov.uk

North Western Deanery
University of Manchester
Dept of Postgraduate Medicine and Dentistry
4th Floor
Barlow House
Minshall Street
Manchester M1 3DZ
Tel.: 0161 237 3690
http://www.nwpgmd.nhs.uk

Oxford Deanery
The Department of Postgraduate Medical & Dental Education
The Triangle Roosevelt Drive, Headington, Oxford OX3 7XP
Tel.: 01865 740 656
http://www.oxford-pgmde.co.uk

Scotland

East Region Office

Tel.: 01382 496516

North Region Office

Tel.: 01224 554365

West Region Office

Tel.: 0141 223 1400

South-East Region

Tel.: 0131 650 2609

http://www.nes.scot.nhs.uk

Severn Institute

Academic Centre

Frenchay Hospital

Frenchay Park Road, Bristol, BS16 1LE

Tel.: 0117 975 7035

http://www.severninstitute.nhs.uk

South West Peninsula Deanery

John Bull Building, Tamar Science Park, Derriford, Plymouth PL6 8BU

Tel.: 01752 437 424

http://www.peninsuladeanery.nhs.uk

South Yorkshire and South Humber
Postgraduate Deans Office

Ground Floor

Don Valley House

Saville Street East

Sheffield S4 7UQ

Tel.: 0114 226 4419

http://www.syshdeanery.com

Wales

Wales School of Postgraduate Medical and Dental Education

University of Wales

College of Medicine

Heath Park

Cardiff CF14 4XN

Tel.: 029 2074 2555 (ST queries)

Tel.: 029 2074 2948/ 3404 (FY queries)

http://www.mmcwales.org

West Midlands Deanery

Institute of Research and Development

Birmingham Research Park

Vincent Drive
Edgbaston
Birmingham B15 2SQ
Tel.: 0121 695 2222
http://www.wmdeanery.org

Yorkshire Deanery
The Dept for NHS Postgraduate Medical and Dental Education
Yorkshire Deanery
University of Leeds
Willow Terrace Road
Leeds LS2 9JT
Tel.: 0113 343 1557
http://www.yorkshiredeanery.com

Disabled Children and Parents

Contact a Family
Supports families with disabled children.
Tel.: 0808 808 3555 (Monday–Friday 10 a.m.–4 p.m., Monday evening 5.30 p.m.–7.30 p.m.)
http://www.cafamily.org.uk

Crossroads
For advice and support if your child has complex needs.
Tel.: 0845 450 0350
http://www.crossroads.org.uk

Disability Benefits Helpline
Tel.: 08457 123 456

Disability Rights Commission
For guidance on legal requirements.
Tel.: 08457 622633

Disabled Parents' Network
Tel.: 0870 241 0450
Email: Information@disabledparentsnetwork.com

Down's Syndrome Association
Tel.: 0845 2300372
http://www.downs-syndrome.org.uk

Early Support Programme
A government initiative to improve services for disabled children and their families, especially those under the age of 5.
Tel.: 0845 60 222 60
http://www.earlysupport.org.uk

Fathers

HomeDad
Supports fathers who stay at home to raise their children.
http://www.homedad.org.uk

Health: You

Action on Pre-Eclampsia (APEC)
Tel.: 020 8427 4217

Association for Postnatal Illness
25 Jerdan Place
London SW6 1BE
Tel.: 020 7386 0868
http://www.apni.org

BMA Counselling Line
Tel.: 08459 200 169 (24 hours)

The Centre for Pregnancy Nutrition
Free leaflets on healthy eating before, during and after pregnancy.
Tel.: 0845 130 3646
http://www.shef.ac.uk/pregnancy_nutrition/

CRY-SIS
Support for families with excessive crying, sleepless, and demanding babies.
Helpline: 08451 228 669
Seven days a week, 9 a.m.–10 p.m.

Doctors' Support Line (for doctors or medical students)
Confidential peer support line staffed by trained volunteer doctors.
Tel.: 0870 765 0001 6pm–11pm Mon–Fri, 10am–11pm Sunday
http://www.doctorssupport.org

Doctors Support Network
Self-help group for doctors with mental illnesses.
Tel.: 0870 321 0 642 (evenings and weekends)
http://www.dsn.org.uk

Infertility Network UK
Charter House
43 St Leonard's Road
Bexhill on sea
East Sussex TN40 1JA
Tel.: 08701 188088
http://www.infertilitynetworkuk.com

The Marcè Society
Mental health support for babies and their mothers.
PO Box 7110, Derby, DE1 0BG, UK
Email: info@marcesociety.com
http://www.marcesociety.com

Medical Sickness Society (MSS)
Tel.: 0808 100 1884
http://www.medical-sickness.co.uk

Miscarriage Association
c/o Clayton Hospital
Northgate
Wakefield
West Yorkshire WF1 3JS
Tel.: 01924 200 799
Fax: 01924 298 834
Email: miscarriageassociation@care4free.net
http://www.miscarriageassociation.org.uk

National AIDS Helpline
Tel.: 0800 567 123 (24 hours)
http://www.condomessentialwear.co.uk

Postnatal illness support group
Helpline with 24-hour answerphone.
Room 18, Stricklandgate House
Stricklandgate
Kendal LA9 4PU
Tel.: 01539 733 893 (Helpline)
http://www.mbha.nhs.uk/mentalhealth/Postnatal

Samaritans
Tel.: 08457 90 90 90

Stillbirth and Neonatal Death Society (SANDS)
Helpline: 020 7436 5881 (10.00 a.m.–5.30 p.m., Monday–Friday)

General enquiries: 020 7436 7940
http://www.uk-sands.org

The Vegetarian Society: A Free Fact sheet
Guide to Nutrition during Pregnancy
Send an SAE to: The Vegetarian Society
Parkdale
Dunham Road
Altrincham
Cheshire. WA14 4QG
Tel.: 0161 925 2000
http://www.vegsoc.org

Health: Babies

BLISS
For parents of premature babies.
Tel.: 0500 618 140
http://www.bliss.org.uk

Cleft Lip and Palate Association (CLAPA)
Tel.: 020 7833 4883
http://www.clapa.com
Email: info@clapa.com

FSID (The Foundation for the Study of Infant Deaths)
Artillery House
11–19 Artillery Row
London SW1P 1RT
Tel.: 020 7233 2090
http://www.fsid.org.uk

Legal advice, rights, and benefits

Advisory, Conciliation and Arbitration Service (ACAS)
For information on employment rights.
Tel.: 0845 747 4747
http://www.acas.org.uk

British Medical Association (BMA)
BMA House
Tavistock Square
London WC1H 9JP
Ask BMA (members only) 0870 60 60 828
http://www.bma.org.uk

Child Benefit Office
PO Box 1
Newcastle upon Tyne NE88 1AA
0845 302 1444 (Great Britain)
0845 603 2000 (Northern Ireland)
http://www.hmrc.gov.uk/childbenefit

Citizens Advice Bureaux
http://www.adviceguide.org.uk

Department of Trade and Industry (DTI)
Tel.: 020 7215 5000
Publications order line: 0845 015 0010
http://www.dti.gov.uk

Department for Work and Pensions
Tel.: 020 7712 2171
http://www.dwp.gov.uk

Employment Tribunals Service
Tel.: 0845 7959 775
http://www.employmenttribunals.gov.uk

Equal Opportunities Commission
Arndale House
Arndale Centre
Manchester M4 3EQ
Tel.: 0845 601 5901 (England)
Tel.: 029 2034 3552 (Wales)
Tel.: 0845 601 5901 (Scotland)
http://www.eoc.org.uk

General Medical Council (GMC)
5th Floor
St James's Buildings
79 Oxford Street
Manchester M1 6FQ
Tel.: 0845 357 8001
http://www.gmc-uk.org

Health and Safety Executive (HSE)
Tel.: 0845 345 0055
http://www.hse.gov.uk

Inland Revenue: for copies of information leaflets
Tel.: 0845 9000 404

Fax: 0845 9000 604
http://www.inlandrevenue.gov.uk

Jobcentre Plus
http://www.jobcentreplus.gov.uk

Know your Rights
For information on workplace issues.
Tel.: 0870 600 4882
http://www.tuc.org.uk

Law Centres
Can sometimes provide advice and free representation in the employment tribunal.
http://www.lawcentres.org.uk

Medical Defence Union (MDU)
230 Blackfriar's Road
London SE1 8PJ
Tel.: 020 7202 1500
http://www.the-mdu.com

The Medical and Dental Defence Union of Scotland
Mackintosh House
120 Blythswood Street
Glasgow G2 4EA
Tel.: 0141 221 5858
Fax: 0141 228 1208
http://www.mddus.com

Medical Protection Society (MPS)
Granary Wharf House
Leeds LS11 5PY
Tel.: 0113 243 6436
Fax: 0113 241 0500
http://www.mps.org.uk

Medical Sickness Society (MSS)
Tel.: 0808 100 1884
http://www.medical-sickness.co.uk

Tax Credits Helpline
Tel.: 0845 300 3900
http://www.hmrc.gov.uk/taxcredits

TIGER (Tailored Interactive Guide on Employment Rights)
http://www.tiger.gov.uk

Working Families

For advice on maternity and paternity rights, and combining work and family.

Tel.: 0800 013 0313 (free legal helpline)

http://www.workingfamilies.org.uk

Maternity wear and children's clothes

Blooming Marvellous

Maternity and babies.

Tel.: 0845 458 7400

http://www.bloomingmarvellous.co.uk

Business Bump/Crave Maternity wear

Maternity wear for professional women.

Tel.: 0870 240 5476

http://www.businessbump.co.uk

Isabella Oliver

Tel.: 0870 240 7612

http://www.IsabellaOliver.com

Mamas and Papas

Tel.: 0870 830 7700

http://www.mamasandpapas.co.uk

Melba

Maternity active and leisurewear.

Tel.: 020 8347 8811

http://www.melbamaternity.co.uk

Mind The Bump

http://www.mindthebump.co.uk

Email: sales@mindthebump.co.uk

Mini Marvellous

For 2–8 year olds.

Tel.: 0845 458 7409

http://www.minimarvellous.co.uk

Mothercare

Tel.: 08453 304030

http://www.mothercare.com

Seraphine

Tel.: 0870 609 2602

http://www.seraphine.com

Military doctors

Army Information Line
Tel.: 08457 300 111

Directorate of Naval Recruitment
Tel.: 02392 727745
http://www.royal-navy.mod.uk/rnmedical

Officer Recruiting
RHQ Royal Army Medical Corps
Keogh Barracks
Ash Vale
Aldershot GU12 5RQ
http://www.army.mod.uk

Medical Liaison Officer
Directorate of Recruiting Selection (Royal Air Force)
PO Box 1000
Cranwell
Sleaford
Lincolnshire NG34 8GZ
Tel.: 01400 261201, ext. 6811
http://www.raf-careers.com

Multiple births

Twins and Multiple Births Association (TAMBA)
Tel.: 0870 7703305 (Mon–Fri 9.30am–4pm)
http://www.tamba.org.uk

Nappies

The Cloth Nappy Campaign
Tel.: 01245 437318

The National Association of Nappy Services
www.changeanappy.co.uk

Twinkle Twinkle
Advice and assistance on reuseable nappies, and for sales of nappies
Tel.: 0118 969 5550
http://www.twinkleontheweb.co.uk
http://www.howtonappy.co.uk
http://www.chooseanappy.co.uk
The above websites offer information on choosing and using reuseable nappies.

Relationships

RELATE: National Marriage Guidance
www.relate.org.uk

Women's Aid National Domestic Violence Helpline
Tel.: 0808 2000 247 (Freephone 24 hours)

Royal colleges and associations

Association of British Neurologists
Ormond House
4th Floor
27 Boswell Street
London WC1N 3JZ
Tel.: 020 7405 4060
Fax: 020 7405 4070
Email: abn@abnoffice.demon.co.uk

Association of Coloproctology
35–43 Lincoln's Inn Fields
London WC2A 3PN
Tel.: 020 7973 0307
Fax: 020 7430 9235
http://www.acpgbi.org.uk

The Association for Palliative Medicine of Great Britain and Ireland
11 Westwood Road
Southampton SO17 1DL
http://www.palliative-medicine.org

Association of Upper Gastrointestinal Surgeons of Great Britain and Ireland
35–43 Lincoln's Inn Fields
London WC2A 3PN
Tel.: 020 7973 0305
Fax: 020 7430 9235

British Association of Dermatologists
4 Fitzroy Square
London W1P 5HQ
Tel.: 020 7383 0266
Fax: 020 7388 5263
http://www.bad.org.uk

British Association of Oral and Maxillofacial Surgeons
Royal College of Surgeons of England
35–43 Lincoln's Inn Fields

London WC2A 3PN
Tel.: 020 7405 8074
Fax: 020 7430 9997
http://www.baoms.org.uk

British Association of Otolaryngologists
Royal College of Surgeons of England
35–43 Lincoln's Inn Fields
London WC2A 3PN
Tel.: 020 7404 8373
Fax: 020 7404 4200
http://www.entuk.org

British Association of Paediatric Surgeons
Royal College of Surgeons of England
35–43 Lincoln's Inn Fields
London WC2A 3PN
Tel.: 020 7869 6915
Fax: 020 7869 6919
http://www.baps.org.uk

British Association of Surgical Oncology
Royal College of Surgeons of England
35–43 Lincoln's Inn Fields
London WC2A 3PN
Tel.: 020 7405 5612
Fax: 020 7404 6574
http://www.baso.org.uk

British Geriatrics Society
31 St John's Square
London EC1M 4DN
Tel.: 020 7608 1369
Fax: 020 7608 1041
http://www.bgs.org.uk

British Orthopaedic Association
Royal College of Surgeons of England
35–43 Lincoln's Inn Fields
London WC2A 3PN
Tel.: 020 7405 6507
Fax: 020 7831 2676
http://www.boa.ac.uk

British Society of Gastroenterologists
3 St Andrew's Place
Regents Park

London NW1 4LB
Tel.: 020 7935 2815
Fax: 020 7487 3734
http://www.bsg.org.uk

The British Society for Rheumatology
Bride House
18–20 Bride Lane
London EC4Y 8EE
Tel.: 020 7842 0900
Fax: 020 7842 0901
http://www.rheumatology.org.uk

Faculty of Accident and Emergency Medicine
Royal College of Physicians
11 St Andrews Place
Regents Park
London NW1 4LE
Tel.: 020 7404 1999

Faculty of Public Health Medicine
Royal College of Physicians
4 St Andrew's Place
London NW1 4LB
Tel.: 020 7935 0243
Fax: 020 7224 6973

Medical Society for the Study of Venereal Diseases
Royal Society of Medicine
1 Wimpole Street
London W1M 8AE
Tel.: 020 7290 2900
Fax: 020 7290 2989
http://www.mssvd.org.uk

Royal College of Anaesthetists
Churchill House
35 Red Lion Square
London WC1R 4SG
Tel.: 020 7092 1500
Fax: 020 7092 1730
http://www.rcoa.ac.uk

Royal College of General Practitioners
14 Prince's Gate

London SW7 1PU
Tel.: 020 7581 3232
Fax: 020 7225 3047
http://www.rcgp.org.uk

Royal College of Obstetricians and Gynaecologists
27 Sussex Place
Regent's Park
London NW1 4RG
Tel.: 020 7772 6200
http://www.rcog.org.uk

Royal College of Ophthalmologists
17 Cornwall Terrace
London NW1 4QW
Tel.: 020 7935 0702
Fax: 020 7935 9838
http://www.rcophth.ac.uk

Royal College of Paediatrics and Child Health
50 Hallum Street
London W1W 6DE
Tel.: 020 7307 5600
Fax: 020 7307 5601
http://www.rcpch.ac.uk

Royal College of Pathologists
2 Carlton House Terrace
London SW1Y 5AF
Tel.: 020 7930 5861
Fax: 020 7321 0523
http://www.rcpath.org

Royal College of Physicians
11 St Andrew's Place
Regent's Park
London NW1 4LE
Tel.: 020 7935 1174
Fax: 020 7487 5218
http://www.rcplondon.ac.uk

Royal College of Physicians and Surgeons of Glasgow
232–242 St Vincent Street
Glasgow G2 5RJ

Tel.: 0141 221 6072
Fax: 0141 221 1804
http://www.rcpsg.ac.uk

Royal College of Psychiatrists
17 Belgrave Square
London SW1X 8PG
Tel.: 020 7235 2351
Fax: 020 7245 1231
http://www.rcpsych.ac.uk

Royal College of Radiologists
38 Portland Place
London W1N 4JQ
Tel.: 020 7636 4432
Fax: 020 7323 3100
http://www.rcr.ac.uk

Royal College of Surgeons of Edinburgh
Nicolson Street
Edinburgh EH8 9DW
Tel.: 0131 527 1600
Fax: 0131 557 6406
http://www.rcsed.ac.uk

Royal College of Surgeons of England
35/43 Lincoln's Inn Fields
London WC2A 3PN
Tel.: 020 7405 3474
Fax: 020 7831 9438
http://www.rcseng.ac.uk

Royal College of Surgeons of Ireland
123 St Stephen's Green
Dublin 2
Tel.: 00 353 1 402 2100
http://www.rcsi.ie

Society of Cardiothoracic Surgeons of Great Britain and Ireland
Royal College of Surgeons of England
35–43 Lincoln's Inn Fields
London WC2A 3PN
Tel.: 020 7405 3474
Fax: 020 7831 9438
http://www.scts.org

Single parents

Child Support Agency
Tel.: 0845 713 3133
http://www.csa.gov.uk

National Council for One Parent Families
Tel.: 0800 018 5026
http://www.oneparentfamilies.org.uk

New Deal for Lone Parents
Tel.: 0800 868 868
http://www.jobcentreplus.gov.uk

One Parent Families/Gingerbread
Tel.: 0800 018 5026 (Mon–Fri 9 a.m.–5 p.m.)
http://www.oneparentfamilies.org.uk

Single Parent Travel Club
6 Bentfield Road
Stansted Mount
Essex CM24 8HW
Tel.: 0870 2416 210
http://www.geocities.com/singleparenttravelclub

Smoking: help with stopping

NHS Smoking Helpline
Tel.: 0800 169 0 169
http://www.gosmokefree.co.uk

Quit
Tel.: 0800 00 22 00 (9 a.m.–9 p.m.)
http://www.quit.org.uk

General

General Medical Council (GMC)
5th Floor
St James's Buildings
79 Oxford Street
Manchester M1 6FQ
Tel.: 0845 357 8001
Fax: 0845 357 9001
Email: gmc@gmc-uk.org
http://www.gmc-uk.org

Medical Women's Federation
Tavistock House North
Tavistock Square
London WC1H 9HX
Tel.: 020 7387 7765
http://www.medicalwomensfederation.org.uk

National Childbirth Trust (NCT)
Alexandra House
Oldham Terrace
London W3 6NH
Tel.: 0870 444 8707
Email: enquiries@national-childbirth-trust.co.uk
http://www.nctpregnancyandbabycare.com

Parentline Plus
For support, information, advice or counseling on many aspects of parenting.
Tel.: 0808 8002 222 (helpline)
http://www.parentlineplus.org.uk

Student Loans Company Ltd
100 Bothwell Street
Glasgow G2 7JD
Tel.: 0870 606 0704

Women in Surgery, WINS (formerly Women in Surgical Training, WIST)
The Royal College of Surgeons of England
35–43 Lincoln's Inn Fields
London WC2A 3PN
Tel.: 020 7869 6212
Fax: 020 7831 9438
http://www.rcseng.ac.uk/career

Working families
1–3 Berry Street
London EC1V 0AA
Tel.: 020 7253 7243
Tel.: 0800 013 0313 (Free legal helpline)
Email: office@workingfamilies.org.uk
http://www.workingfamilies.org.uk

The Good Birth Company
Birth pool hire.
Tel.: 0800 035 0514
http://www.thegoodbirth.co.uk

Index